Last Drinks

How to drink less and be your best

Maz Compton

WILEY

First published in 2023 by John Wiley & Sons Australia, Ltd
Level 4, 600 Bourke St, Melbourne, Victoria 3000, Australia

Typeset in Adobe Jenson Pro 11.5pt/15.5pt

© Super Rad Productions Pty Ltd 2023

The moral rights of the author have been asserted

ISBN: 978-1-394-18423-1

NATIONAL LIBRARY OF AUSTRALIA

A catalogue record for this book is available from the National Library of Australia

Cover design by Alissa Dinalo
Figure 2.2: Image: © ttsz/Getty Images
Figure 2.3: Image: © Blamb/Shutterstock
Printed and bound by CPI Group (UK) Ltd, Croydon, CR0 4YY

Disclaimer
The material in this publication is of the nature of general comment only, and does not represent professional advice. It is not intended to provide specific guidance for particular circumstances and it should not be relied on as the basis for any decision to take action or not take action on any matter which it covers. Readers should obtain professional advice where appropriate, before making any such decision. To the maximum extent permitted by law, the author and publisher disclaim all responsibility and liability to any person, arising directly or indirectly from any person taking or not taking action based on the information in this publication.

C9781394184231_120623

Contents

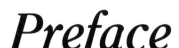

Preface

The term 'sober curious' — choosing to avoid alcohol for personal or wellness reasons — didn't exist in 2015 when I started my sobriety journey. The brilliant and articulate — *cough* — way people reacted when I told them I was 'just not drinking right now' included …

'You're what?'

'Get f**ked Compton?'

'When did you become so boring?'

'Call me when you get back on that wagon.'

None of this was helpful.

I wasn't chaotic. Nothing terrible happened. I didn't do anything outrageously ridiculous. I just wanted to dance until the break of dawn and sometimes I'd overshare on Twitter. From the outside looking in, I was functioning. I was fine. My unravelling was slow and steady. In fact, I thought my story was quite unique. I wanted to stop drinking and I had no idea how to, so I kept drinking, always hoping the next day would be different. But it wasn't.

As it turns out, my story isn't unique; it's everywhere. Each day was a murkier version of the previous one. I was caught in a battle between two voices in my head: the voice that begged me to stop drinking, and the voice that shouted louder, frustrated at the thought of needing to stop, because if I needed to stop and couldn't, then maybe I did have a drinking problem after all. Sound familiar?

In her book *The Lies About Truth*, Courtney C Stevens wisely writes, 'If nothing changes, nothing changes. If you keep doing what you're doing, you're going to keep getting what you're getting. You want change, make some.' I kept carrying out the same behaviour and expecting a different result. I kept drinking and hoping to feel better, to find peace, to be able to relax, for the anxiety to dissipate. But the blame-shame cycle ended up driving me slightly batty. I was doing my own head in. For things to change, guess what? Something needed to change. So, I made the brave, bold decision to change my drinking behaviour, just for a month, to see what was on the other side of my last drink. And it turns out, that was an excellent decision. By redefining my relationship with alcohol, I redesigned my life.

My last drink

My last drink was on New Year's Eve, 2014. It was at the end of a very long New Year's Eve lunch that peaked with my polishing off a bottle of champers with my boyfriend. Perfectly positioned under the Sydney Harbour Bridge at a VIP party. Baby, you're a firework. From what I remember, we had a good time. Getting home from the city with tens of thousands of other enthused and boozed party people was, from what I remember, frustrating. We eventually caught a taxi and crashed at a hotel in the early hours of a new year. Oh, what a night. We woke up at lunch time and ate pizza.

Triple cheese. Thanks for asking.

My first day of sobriety was relatively easy. Holed up in a fancy hotel with the air-conditioning on 21 degrees Celsius, ordering room service, afternoon catnapping and binge-watching Netflix. We had nowhere to be and nothing to do. Happy New Year. The next day was similar, but it started with a morning ocean swim. I'd just relocated to Sydney from Melbourne to start a new job and along with the move for an amazing career opportunity came the evolution of my relationship status from long-distance to the post-honeymoon phase of our courtship.

Those first two days of sobriety were a cinch, and then it was really really hard.

But I did it.

And I haven't had a drink since.

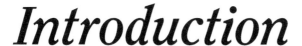

Introduction

For the most part, my adult life was one big manifestation of greatness, but my world spun on an axis where everything involved alcohol. I remember thinking to myself in 2014, 'How can anyone exist in a world obsessed with alcohol, without alcohol?' That was my year of sober curiosity and the final year I drank alcohol. At the time though, not drinking seemed like a terrifying thought, an outrageous, rebellious act, an impossible quest.

In 2014 I drank ... a lot. What's a lot, you ask? Most days, a bottle of wine, sometimes more. You know, all the stereotypical incidents depicted in the movies about 'raging alcoholics'. People who are out of control, who have major drinking problems. They act out, end up in prison, ruin their families and for some reason they don't seem to have shoes. Well, none of that happened to me. I had my life in check. I had plenty of shoes. My drinking habits didn't find a rock-bottom moment. I didn't hurt anyone or do anything crazy.

You see, I was working in my dream job in media, living in a dream town in Melbourne and I had met my dreamy future husband that same year. It was all good — at least on paper. And so, yes,

I drank a lot. So what? I drank after work, but never in the morning. I always got myself home safely after a night out, and even though I sometimes didn't remember the taxi ride home, I was okay, so it was okay. Right? I had these invisible boundaries to help prove to myself, and anyone who asked, that I didn't have 'a drinking problem'. No-one wants to admit they have 'a problem' with anything, especially alcohol and especially me.

Is this story starting to feel familiar?

In 2014, towards the winter, I started going out less, and staying in more, but I kept up my daily quota of empty calories by drinking. After work I'd go to a hip-hop yoga class or maybe the gym, drive home via the drive-thru bottle shop, and buy a bottle of Sauvignon Blanc and a Pinot, just in case. I'd walk through my front door — brown paper bags under one arm, handbag in the other — kick off my fabulous shoes, undo my bra strap, sigh loudly and pour a glass of wine. I would finish the bottle while I did normal stuff like shower, cook or order dinner, and decompress from the day. At some point I'd get myself into bed and fall asleep. My apartment was my sanctuary, a place where I could hide away and relax, and the wine helped. Sometimes I'd leave the heater on. Sometimes I'd sleep in my clothes. Usually I'd wake in the middle of the night, have some water, change into my pyjamas and go back to sleep only to wake up minutes later needing to pee. This was my routine. This was my normal. The next day I would get up, shake it off, start again, try again, say I wasn't going to drink again, go to work and begin the cycle again.

I had a busy radio job, one that I love love loved! I hosted the National Drive Show in 2014. I had an excellent executive producer, and an extraordinarily demanding work schedule. You see, I had to keep it together. I couldn't have a problem. I didn't have time for that. If people found out, it would be my undoing: the shame, the judgement, the headlines. The fear of my drinking secret being exposed crippled me into hiding it — my secret shame. To feel like I had control in my over-planned and structured-to-the-microsecond schedule, I drank. At least I could control that...until I couldn't anymore.

You see, I didn't have a problem with alcohol.

Alcohol was the problem.

My relationship with alcohol had become problematic.

In 2015, I embarked on a month-long self-experiment, a very casual stroll into sobriety. I had been questioning my drinking behaviour for years. It was clear I had developed a dependence. I didn't hit rock-bottom; I arrived at a crossroads.

If you have picked up this book, or it has been carefully placed in an obvious location in your house by a loved one, you too might be questioning your relationship with alcohol. That's okay. I've been there: it's called 'sober curiosity' and no, there isn't anything wrong with you. Somehow your relationship with alcohol is out of balance. It's having a negative effect despite your best efforts to keep a handle on it. You can function, right? You get by okay. But there is a voice in your very busy head questioning if maybe you need to stop. And you have no idea how to.

And aren't you exhausted?

I was.

I was so exhausted.

On paper my life looked like a dream, but in the privacy of my tiny apartment in Melbourne, I was living in a nightmare. You might be able to relate to that — you might be disliking your situation as much as I did.

Thriving without alcohol

This book is designed as a guide to help you discover a new approach to life, one where you are free from alcohol. It showcases how you can live a sober life and love it. I wrote this book to help you solve the internal conflict that you are tired of hearing on repeat and to equip you with practical tools for thriving without alcohol, so you can create a life that loves you back and showers you with inner peace. A life without alcohol will lead to your happiest and healthiest days. Now, can you please do me a favour? Can you please take everything you think you know about alcohol, your relationship with it and what it does for you, and in your mind place a big fat question mark there so we can explore the other side of what you think you know? Keep an open mind.

Can you do that? Yes, yes you can.

This book has been curated with the clear intention of helping you rediscover your strength. It's time for you to rewrite your own rulebook about alcohol and take flight into a new season of life. Included are inspiring stories of overcoming alcohol, embracing sobriety, hearts being healed and purpose being birthed, as well as alcohol facts and stats presented by several experts in their field.

In the pages of this book, you'll find sobriety stories, which are excerpts from some of the conversations I have engaged with on my podcast, 'Last Drinks'. Full episodes are referenced in 'Your Sober Toolkit' at the back of the book should you wish to listen to them. The stories presented about alcohol and sobriety are reinforced with these candid, honest, real stories.

In addition you'll have an opportunity to curate your personal Sober Toolkit, which will equip you with tools to set you up for successfully achieving sobriety. Along with this I've included activities that will help you discover a clear intention for your sobriety.

Congratulations on your bold choice to begin a process of self-learning, awareness and change for your own betterment. There is a saying, mostly attributed to Buddha, that states, 'When the student is ready, the teacher will appear'. I believe this to be most appropriate when tapping into sobriety, and a key concept to keep in mind when assessing change management. As a student of sobriety, you will find lots of learning, exploration, uncovering and growing. So many wonderful and challenging things lie ahead. Welcome to the adventure.

Disclaimer: *The doctors consulted for this book are medical professionals. However, it is advisable to seek an appointment with a medical professional for your personal circumstances. The advice offered in this book is general.*

Part I

The truth about alcohol

In part I we'll get a clear understanding of alcohol by defining terms associated with alcohol, exploring scientific facts about the role alcohol plays in our morbidity—as well as its impact on people and society—and identifying some key behaviours associated with drinking.

1 Alcohol is the problem

In this chapter I will put together the case for why alcohol is the problem. There is a stigma attached to narratives about alcohol in our lives: denial, downplaying and deflection. And there is a major oversight when assessing the true and very real effects alcohol has on individuals, families and society at large.

> *Our cultural relationship with alcohol is completely dysfunctional and the amount of trauma, pain, violence and death this drug causes in our community is horrifying. I'm not saying everyone should stop drinking. I would just like us to have a decent conversation about its impacts.*
> **Osher Günsberg — TV and podcast host, sober since 2010**

Our culture has been founded on and built around the consumption of drinks: every emotion on the spectrum, every event on the calendar. There is always an excuse for 'drinks, tipples and drinky-poos'. In our modern-day Western society, drinking is normal. You can smash beer at a BBQ, champers at a celebration, gin after golf, daiquiris after dark. We have pre-mixers, cases, cans and nightcaps. The alcohol industry is worth billions of dollars.

Australia's culture obsession with alcohol can be traced back to the First Fleet. A quick history lesson: when the First Fleet set off from England on 13 May 1787, Arthur Phillip — the first governor of New South Wales — insisted on bringing two years' worth of carefully rationed food for the new settlement, and four years' worth of rum. Our society has long been saturated in booze. In fact, alcohol has been a type of currency in Australia since its earliest documented times so it's no wonder there are groups of people and individuals in our society who are struggling with their relationship with alcohol.

And by 2014, I was one of them.

Alcohol is everywhere

The portrayal of alcohol as necessary for fun times has over-shadowed the truth about alcohol. This has created a narrative that overlooks the dangers of alcohol and its many impacts on individuals and families, and across communities. Drinking too much alcohol can lead to any number of short- and long-term effects, be they physical, emotional, social or mental. In the media industry I saw firsthand how alcohol was the glue for social engagements, launches, press tours, gigs, concerts, events and the wrap party, where everyone could let their hair down after a job well done. It is considered normal to drink to mark the joy of a good day, the middle of a long day, the end of a bad day, a Monday-to-Friday or a Saturday-and-Sunday. Our social interactions go hand in hand with an expectation of alcohol at every gathering, despite the depth and range of adverse impacts alcohol causes.

Sometimes when I drank, I would only have a few drinks; other times I would drink the bar dry. My hangovers would range anywhere from bearable to barely able to open my eyes. In my 20s a beer would give me a buzz, but when I was closer to midlife, I needed a bottle of wine to get the same feeling. As my tolerance for alcohol increased, my bounce-back bottomed out. Over time my relationship with alcohol shifted from tolerable to total train-wreck. Drinking became how I engaged in my entire life. It's how I was able to exist in the world I created, and it felt totally normal.

> We live in a more understanding society. There is a level of acceptance now about sobriety and things are changing with the sober curious movement. People are more understanding of why people are not drinking alcohol.
> **Victoria Vanstone, alcohol-free living advocate**

At first glance, drinking behaviours in society are categorised in a very black-and-white way: either normal and inconsequential or abnormal and consequential. Someone's drinking is either carefree with zero negative effects or uncontrollable and dangerous. Not for me though. I was very much in the grey area of the spectrum of drinking behaviour: it wasn't working for me, but it wasn't ruining my life.

Some facts about alcohol

Consider these facts about how alcohol affects our health and life that you might not be aware of:

- Alcohol kills one person every 10 seconds worldwide.
- Alcohol is classified as a Group 1 carcinogen by the World Health Organization (WHO).
- Alcohol is linked to 5.3 per cent of deaths worldwide, or approximately 3 million people a year.
- Alcohol is a causal factor in more than 200 disease and injury conditions.

Let's take a closer look at what alcohol is and how it can impact us.

What is alcohol?

Put simply, alcohol is a poison. Alcohol refers to a variety of drinks, including but not limited to beer, wine or spirits, that contain a chemical known as ethyl alcohol, or ethanol. Yes — that's the same stuff that you put in your car. In its simplest explanation, alcohol is a mood-changing substance that can be categorised in the 'depressant' category of drugs. Yes — it is a drug. A depressant doesn't directly cause depression; however, it slows down and inhibits the central nervous system. According to healthdirect, for some people depression can be a mood side-effect linked to alcohol consumption.

What does alcohol do?

Alcohol has myriad negative impacts. It has been proven to have significant negative impacts on society and the economy. Once consumed, alcohol can cause havoc on a person, impacting mental and physical health, as well as on relationships and cognitive function. Alcohol is a psychoactive substance with dependence-producing properties, and it can cause many different diseases.

How does alcohol affect the body?

Did you know that alcohol isn't digested in the body? When you have a drink, the alcohol passes quickly into your bloodstream and travels to every part of your body. Alcohol affects your brain first, then your kidneys, lungs and liver. Its effect on your body depends on your age, gender, weight and the type and amount of alcohol consumed. It will generally take your body an hour to break down the alcohol content of one standard drink. And, in case you were wondering, vomiting, taking a cold shower or having a coffee doesn't remove alcohol from your system.

It will generally take your body an hour to break down the alcohol content of one standard drink.

What is grey area drinking?

A grey area drinker is someone who drinks too much, too often. They are usually acutely aware that their drinking behaviour is having some form of negative impact on their life in a physical or mental health capacity, in their relationships or otherwise, but they aren't physically dependent on alcohol. They drink by choice, not to avoid withdrawal symptoms. Grey area drinkers can usually stop drinking if they want to — for a while — but fall back into the cycle of drinking after some time. Accompanying grey area drinking behaviour is an internal dialogue around drinking and whether it's problematic enough that you need to stop. Grey area drinkers are also known as social drinkers, and over time their alcohol tolerance will increase.

What is binge drinking?

Binge drinking is a style of drinking, usually done in social groups, where a lot of drinks are consumed in a short period of time. Most people who binge drink don't have a severe alcohol use disorder (which I will describe shortly). The Centers for Disease Control and Prevention defines binge drinking as the consumption of five or more standard drinks on any one occasion for men, or four or more standard drinks on any one occasion for women. Binge drinkers find themselves drinking to excess with the effects including vomiting, risky behaviour, passing out, decreased cognitive functionality and memory loss.

> *The term 'binge drinking' means different things to different people. Most people agree that a binge would be a session where you deliberately drink to get drunk. For some it's when usually responsible 'light' drinkers overindulge — even just a little. But when we look at the guidelines, it's simply when you consume more than four drinks in any one day.*
> **Dr Sam Hay, GP**

What is alcohol use disorder (AUD)?

Alcohol use disorder (AUD) is a medical condition characterised by an inability to stop drinking or control alcohol consumption despite its negative impacts on an individual — be these social, physical, mental or otherwise. This definition encompasses the drinking behaviours referred to as alcohol abuse, alcohol misuse, alcohol dependence, alcohol addiction and the colloquial (and outdated) term, alcoholism. AUD is considered by health professionals to be a brain disorder ranging from mild to moderate or severe. The lasting changes alcohol misuse can cause in the brain can make an individual susceptible to relapsing. However, there is some good news according to the National Institute on Alcohol Abuse and Alcoholism (NIAAA): no matter how severe the alcohol use problem, evidence-based treatment with behavioural therapies, mutual-support groups and/or medications can assist people in overcoming AUD to achieve and maintain sobriety.

What is 'hangxiety'?

Hangxiety isn't a formal term or diagnosis, but there are plenty of people who identify with the feeling. It's waking up — usually around 3 am — after a big night of drinking and experiencing a hangover with heightened feelings of shame and anxiety.

> If it were discovered tomorrow, there's no way we would allow alcohol to be legal. It is a drug... you can walk into a bottle shop today and buy enough gin to kill you, and it's completely legal. I'm not okay with that. This drug is incredibly destructive. Not everyone reacts to alcohol the way I do, but there are enough people in our community that react badly to alcohol that we should have a good look at it.
>
> **Osher Günsberg — TV and podcast host, sober since 2010**

Summing up ...

+ Alcohol is the problem.

+ Alcohol is a poison. It is highly addictive and perfectly legal, and it can have many negative impacts and downsides for both individuals and society at large.

+ Our society is set up to have alcohol at every engagement and this can be traced back to colonial times.

+ There are many terms associated with drinking behaviour including grey area drinking, binge drinking, alcohol use disorder and 'hangxiety'.

+ By exploring what alcohol is, how it impacts us and why our society is alcohol obsessed, we can gain a new perspective about alcohol and understand our relationship with it better.

Perhaps for you, alcohol is like what it was for me: a daily habit that started out innocently as a social norm and became a part of who you are. It is your way of coping with social engagements, work demands and family pressures, and it is considered normal by your peers.

Now that you have a better understanding of alcohol and how it is impacting your life and relationships, let's dig a little deeper and drill down on what alcohol can do to our brains, our bodies and our behaviours.

2 The impacts of alcohol

Let's take a closer look at the impacts alcohol can have across a variety of measures. This information is factual, grounded in science and presented by a team of experts in their given fields. It is important to understand this information to help you identify and resolve your relationship with alcohol. The World Health Foundation has reported that there is no safe level of alcohol consumption. Just to be clear, the brainiest researchers in the world on health have concluded, with no mincing of words, that *alcohol is not safe for human consumption.*

> *I have many patients who constantly gauge their consumption on what is 'sociably acceptable', often drinking at that level many days a week, unaware of the significant harm they are enduring as they drink at a level significantly above the guidelines.*
> **Dr Sam Hay, GP**

Alcohol and you

Alcohol causes a wide range of problems for a wide range of people and is among the leading preventable risk factors for both physical and social harms globally. An international study at the University of Washington led by the Institute for Health Metrics and Evaluation (IHME), the results of which were published in *The Lancet,* suggests people under 40 should not drink alcohol, stating there were no health benefits from drinking alcohol, only risks for adults aged 15 to 39.

Figure 2.1 illustrates how our thoughts can trigger feelings, which can impact our behaviours, and the order of triggers and impacts are interchangeable, whether they be positive or negative.

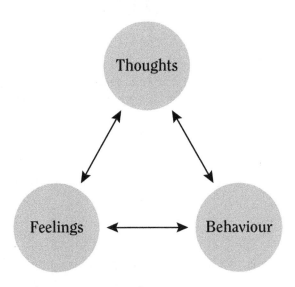

Figure 2.1: the cognitive triangle

Alcohol and your brain

There is no safe amount of alcohol consumption for the brain. Alcohol is a toxin to brain cells and at any level can increase the risk of dementia and the risk of alcohol-related brain damage.
Dr Buddhi Lokuge, addiction expert, PhD, MD

Alcohol consumption can change your brain chemistry, resulting in decreased memory and impaired judgement. According to a 2021 study published in the journal *Scientific Reports*, people with AUD have less brain matter than people without AUD.

What does this mean?

Well, the affected brain areas control a range of important skills including attention, language, memory and reasoning. A 2021 study of more than 25 000 people in the UK found that a moderate consumption of alcohol can adversely affect almost every part of your brain. The study, which is still to be peer-reviewed, suggests that the more alcohol consumed, the lower the brain volume. In effect, the more you drink, the worse off your brain is. Other studies, such as one discussed in the journal *Neurology* in 2014, validate this suggestion by agreeing that alcohol can impact memory and heavy drinkers are at risk of memory loss, experiencing cognitive decline up to six year earlier than non-drinkers.

An expert in the field

Dr Ineka Whiteman

As a doctor of neuroscience, Dr Ineka Whiteman is passionate about helping people understand the science of the brain, mind and body; the inextricable relationship between them; and the practical ways we can nourish, enrich and harness their potential.

Here's what I discovered during my podcast interview with Dr Ineka.

The brain relies on a balance of chemicals and processes to function. Alcohol consumption affects different parts of the brain.

Our thinking and our behaviour are intrinsically linked, and this sentiment is grounded in science. When we look at the brain, it's good to look at a microscopic level: it's a

(continued)

fleshy lump of tissue that sits inside our skull made up of more than 100 billion neurons (brain cells). The neurons are incredibly small, but these tiny cells are little powerhouses that enables all the different functions of our brain, including our thoughts, emotions, learning, memory and formation of habits (both good and bad!).

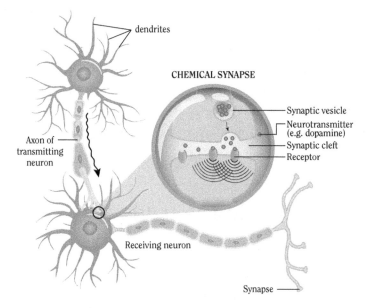

Figure 2.2: how neurons communicate

How do thoughts occur?

Let's have a look at figure 2.2 and how neurons enable us to have and process thoughts. We can think of neurons like billions of tiny chia seeds making up the fleshy substance of our brain (although they are in fact much smaller than chia seeds, you can fit about 50 neurons across the width of a human hair). Each of these tiny seeds grows 'arms', called dendrites and a long axon which acts like an insulated electrical cord, carrying signals from one end of the cell to the other.

Each individual neuron can connect and receive signals from up to 7000 other neurons, making highly complex 'neural networks' throughout our brain.

Neurons communicate through sending 'electrochemical' signals to each other. When we have a thought, for example, a neuron generates an electrical charge which travels down the axon at about 100m/sec until it reaches the end of the axon. There we see a gap between neurons known as the 'synapse'. To transmit the signal across this synapse, the electrical signal stimulates the release of 'vesicles' or tiny sacs of chemicals called neurotransmitters, which float across the synapse and are taken up by specialised receptors on the dendrites of the 'receiving neuron' on the other side. This chemical signal is then converted into an electrical signal which travels along the neuron, hits the synapse triggering a chemical signal, and so on and so on. This creates a process of 'electro-chemical signalling', which is how a thought travels through our brain.

It's important to know that each time the same thought process occurs, electro-chemical messages cross the same synapse, in the same pathway, strengthening the connection between the communicating neurons. The more times we have the same thought over and over, the stronger that connection between the neurons becomes. As the saying goes, 'neurons that fire together, wire together.' This is the basis of how we learn new things, new skills, form memories and form habits — by practising the same thing over and over we are strengthening the neural pathways right down to the molecular level. On the flip side, neurons that don't communicate with each other will eventually lose those strong connections between them and, with it, those thoughts, habits and skills will fade. This is known as the 'use it or lose it' principal. This powerful,

(continued)

dynamic ability for the brain to change and reorganise itself in response to different inputs is known as neuroplasticity. And this remarkable process is key to the changing of our habits, as we will see later in Chapter 4.

How does alcohol affect our brain?

As we have seen, alcohol is a depressant, which means it can disrupt the chemical balance in our brain, affecting our thoughts, feelings and actions. This is partly due to the changes in the neurotransmitters, which help to transmit communication signals from one neuron to another. Consuming alcohol triggers an immediate release of certain neurochemicals.

When you drink alcohol, two key things then happen:

1. *Gamma-aminobutyric acid (GABA) pathways are activated in your brain.* GABA is the major 'inhibitory' neurotransmitter in the brain, blocking or slowing down electrical signals, and giving us that calm, chilled-out vibe. You know: the relaxed feeling you get from that first sip of wine after work. The alcohol triggers the GABA-related inhibitory pathways in your brain, making you feel this way. However, if you have more than a few glasses of alcohol, the over-activity of the GABA pathways is what leads to clumsiness, slurred speech, loss of balance, slower reaction times and feeling sedated. This perfect storm of feeling relaxed and uninhibited, while also becoming increasingly sluggish and clumsy, is what leads us to do stupid things when we're drunk, like scaling a paddock fence in heels, or worse. Drinking to excess can cause extreme sedation of the brain and central nervous system and, in turn, alcohol toxicity and overdose.

2. *Glutamate and dopamine are activated.* Alcohol speeds up the release of another neurotransmitter called glutamate, which is responsible for regulating the major 'reward' chemical in the brain called dopamine. Deep in our brains is a region known as the ventral tegmental area (VTA), which makes connections to the nucleus accumbens and prefrontal cortex — together, they work together as the 'reward centre' of our brain (see figure 2.3, overleaf). When we drink alcohol, the neurons in the VTA release dopamine onto the nucleus accumbens and we interpret that as 'feeling good'. Even small amounts of alcohol increases dopamine release in the 'reward centre' which leads to that pleasurable 'warm and fuzzy' feeling. Not a bad thing in itself, however this structure of the brain is also the reason why we become addicted to certain pleasures. The more we experience that dopamine release and the feel-good feeling, the more we want that feel-good feeling. So basically, alcohol activates our pleasure centres, gives us that chilled, feel-good buzz: so we keep drinking to feel good. The problem? Well, over time, people who drink regularly begin to notice that one or two glasses of alcohol don't have the same effect on them that it used to. The dopamine receptors in the reward centres start to become desensitised and 'tolerant' of alcohol, which means higher quantities of alcohol are needed to produce the same feel-good effect. And so begins the vicious cycle of needing more and more to feel good, which can eventually lead to alcohol dependence.

(continued)

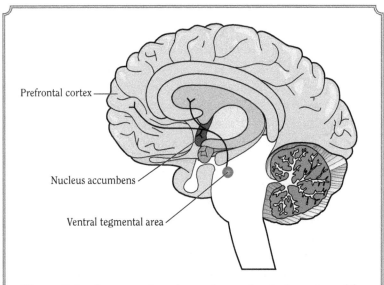

Prefrontal cortex

Nucleus accumbens

Ventral tegmental area

Figure 2.3: the reward pathway in our brain is activated by glutamate and dopamine release when we drink alcohol

What's the good news?

Here are some of the positive things that occur in your brain when you stop drinking alcohol:

+ At first, a lack of dopamine and diminished receptor activation can lead to feelings of sadness, anxiety and irritability. However, over time, without alcohol the brain begins to restore its natural dopamine levels, increasing your ability to feel good again without a substance.

+ Our brain functions are directly impacted by alcohol use, which can have negative impacts on memory and rational thinking. However, over time, new cells and synapse connections will form and can overcome this damage.

- Early sobriety can result in moodiness. Over time, however, as you heal, you will experience a sense of heightened motivation towards more beneficial goals.

- Your emotional regulation will evolve as your brain builds new connections and creates pathways for healthy, positive interactions in the future.

- By eliminating alcohol, you can better understand your mental health and determine what it is you need to feel your best.

- Experiencing life without alcohol means you must learn new coping mechanisms and social skills. This is an opportunity for your brain power to grow and evolve as you begin to engage in the social activities you enjoy, but without alcohol.

- You regain control over your life, choices, behaviours and attitudes.

Alcohol and your body

Alcohol can have a gamut of negative health impacts on the body. Making this even more complex is the fact that alcohol affects everyone differently.

I want to pat my tummy when I think about this, you know when you drink too much, you are often on the toilet, and it's just not great, I realised that was my body reacting to the alcohol, so when I stopped drinking, things settled right down and I found that quite incredible.
Yumi Stynes — media personality and author, sober since 2014

In the short term, drinking too much alcohol can negatively impact many parts of the body — and I'm not just talking about falling down a set of stairs or off a bar stool. Drinking even a small amount of alcohol reduces your body's natural immune system. A weakened immune system has a harder time protecting you from germs and viruses, opening you up to a higher likelihood of getting sick.

Alcohol causes inflammation in the body and can cause the pancreas to produce toxic substances that can lead to dangerous inflammation. Inflammation prevents proper digestion. Over a long period of time, or drinking too much alcohol on a single occasion, can damage your heart leading to complications including high blood pressure and even stroke. Heavy drinking also takes its toll on the liver.

Put simply, the more people drink, the more deadly the effects. There's conclusive evidence that excessive alcohol consumption is associated with higher rates of mortality.
Dr Sam Hay, GP

What's more, long-term alcohol use can affect bone density leading to thinner bones and increasing your risk of fractures. Weakened bones may heal more slowly. Drinking alcohol can also lead to muscle weakness, cramping and, eventually, atrophy. Outside of our internal bodily function, alcohol can lead to unnecessary injury, accidents, self-harm, risky sexual behaviour, violence, alcohol poisoning and hangovers.

When you drink, toxins build up in the deeper layers of your skin. This can manifest as any number, or a combination of, bloating, puffiness, acne, redness, flushing, premature ageing and an increase in wrinkles. Drinking alcohol can lower your inhibitions, and heavy drinking can prevent sex hormone production, lower your libido, keep you from getting or maintaining an erection and make it difficult to achieve orgasm. Excessive drinking may affect your menstrual cycle and potentially increase your risk of infertility. And finally, alcohol is jam-packed full of calories with zero nutrition (that is, empty calories) and can cause weight gain in four ways: it stops your body from burning fat, it's high in kilojoules, it can make you feel hungry and it can lead to poor food choices. In other words, alcohol consumption makes it more challenging to manage your weight effectively.

An expert in the field

Dr Andrew Rochford

As an emergency doctor and media personality, Dr Andrew Rochford has seen firsthand the impact alcohol consumption can have. With a passion for helping people manage the stressors in their lives to find balance and wholeness, Dr Andrew shares his professional insights about alcohol and what it does to the physical body as well as its impact on mental health. Andrew is a national spokesperson for the Australian Digital Health Agency and Drinkwise.

Alcohol wreaks havoc in our bodies. As you drink alcohol, it passes through the walls of the stomach and small intestine into your blood. It then travels to the different parts of your body, affecting all organs, cells and systems. Alcohol affects your brain first. It slows down your thinking, reaction time and decision making. It also impacts the way you feel and behave. Then it affects your lungs, kidney and liver. Once it reaches your liver it is metabolised, or broken down, and removed from the blood stream. Alcohol essentially keeps your body in survival mode. Your physical body and all its complex, interconnected systems can't be in survival mode and repair/rest mode simultaneously; therefore, alcohol keeps your body in a chronic state of stress.

(continued)

Not only does alcohol impact our physical body, add to our sleep debt and in general keep us on the back foot, but it also puts us at risk for many diseases, and can impact our mental health. For some people who experience anxiety, a drink may help them feel more at ease. But this feeling is short-lived. The so-called 'relaxed' feeling we get after having a drink is due to the chemical changes alcohol causes in the brain. These effects wear off fast. Relying on alcohol to mask anxiety could also lead to a greater reliance on it to relax.

Ironically, drinking alcohol can also increase anxiety because when we drink, we don't always respond to all the cues around us. If we're prone to anxiety and notice something that could be interpreted as threatening in the environment, there is a tendency to focus on that and miss the other less threatening — or neutral — information. Excessive alcohol consumption can result in injury, emotional harm and memory loss.

When it comes to sober curiosity, awareness is an important first step. It's the simple recognition that your alcohol consumption is having a negative effect, or that you are drinking more, or more often, than you would like. Becoming aware of and recognising your relationship with alcohol and its impact on you is a good first step to actively changing your drinking behaviour. Asking yourself questions about your drinking may help to identify your current relationship with alcohol. The very questioning of your drinking behaviour is a firm indication that your alcohol consumption may be impacting your life in a negative way.

What's the good news?

Just as there are myriad health impacts alcohol can have on your body, the reverse is also true. Reducing your alcohol consumption can dramatically improve your body's ability to function. Saying no to alcohol is likely to lower your risk of serious diseases such as several types of cancer, heart disease, liver disease, high blood pressure and stroke, and is likely to improve your overall physical and mental health.

The immediate short-term benefits of cutting out alcohol can include:

+ better sleep
+ weight loss
+ lower blood sugar
+ lower blood pressure
+ fewer hangovers and alcohol-related symptoms such as headaches, heartburn, indigestion and stomach upsets
+ less fat build-up around the liver
+ improving existing conditions such as depression, high blood pressure and skin conditions
+ more energy
+ better absorption of nutrients such as vitamins B1 and B12, folic acid and zinc
+ fewer injuries.

In the long term, reducing your alcohol intake reduces the risk of:

+ strokes
+ depression, anxiety and mental health conditions
+ cancer
+ liver disease
+ high blood pressure and cardiac disease
+ many other alcohol-related conditions.

Questionable research seemed to imply that a person could drink a glass of red wine and reap health benefits. These studies have since been criticised for flawed methodology but still used in advocacy for more than a decade. It is irresponsible to promote the idea that there are health benefits to any level of alcohol consumption given the wide ranging harms we know it causes to individuals and population health.
Dr Buddhi Lokuge, addiction expert, PhD, MD

In 2011 I lived in Adelaide for a while. I was post divorce, on an early radio show career trajectory and high functioning, but I had what I considered a quite manageable alcohol dependence. During this time, I visited the local wineries — often — and my left eye kept randomly becoming swollen and itchy. It would flare up overnight and in the morning, unfortunately for my breakfast radio co-hosts, my face resembled a female version of Sloth from *The Goonies*, you know, the 'hey you guys', guy. Red, itchy, swollen, inflamed — you get the picture. It wasn't pretty.

A quick trip to my doctor and a round of steroid cream would bring it under control, but after several visits to the doctor and a few conversations, she suggested I could in fact have an allergy to a particular preservative. After hearing how much red wine I drank at the time, she concluded that I was quite possibly allergic to a preservative found predominantly in red wine.

So, rather than address my relationship with alcohol, I started drinking Sauvignon Blanc.

Alcohol and sleep

Good-quality sleep is essential for our mental, emotional and physical health, and alcohol before bed is a sleep thief, not a sleep aid. So what does alcohol do to our sleep?

I certainly went through a very long season where I would drink to help myself get to sleep. And if I had a big night out, I would wake up at 3 am feeling super anxious. My heart would be racing and my head would be swirling, trying to piece together fragments of the night before.

My mouth would be dry beyond comprehension. My comprehension would be beyond understanding. My understanding of the current situation would be nonexistent. I would wake up with my head pounding, and stumble across the room to guzzle some water and a few aspirins before going back to bed. My sleep was broken. I was at breaking point and yet the days played out like a broken record.

> I had learned over the years to cope with stress and anxiety by drinking wine. I could easily polish off a bottle of red on a weekday to take away the pain of what was really going on, because in that moment I thought the wine was helping. Unfortunately, I would wake up the next morning and my anxiety would be 10 times worse. And so the cycle would continue.
>
> **Heidi Anderson — radio host and author**

Drinking disrupts your sleep cycle. You might think having a good old glass of red before bed will carry you off to the land of nod with ease. In fact, it is very common for people to use alcohol as a sleep aid because of its sedative properties. However, the negative effects on your sleep quality far outweigh the false sense of relaxation and ease that a glass of wine can offer in getting you off to sleep. As the quality of your sleep is impacted negatively by alcohol, you can be left tired and grumpy the next day.

Add to this that you will more than likely wake up with a hangover if you've had a lot to drink. As well as feeling tired and having a headache you may also have feelings of stress and irritability. When you drink alcohol, you may find you have to get up in the night to go to the toilet, further disrupting your sleep cycle. And because alcohol is a diuretic, it encourages the body to lose extra fluid, not only in urine, but also through sweat, making dehydration worse.

Okay, you get the picture.

Let's now cover off some sleep basics.

The sleep cycle

A sleep cycle lasts about 90 minutes. During this time, we move through five stages of sleep. The first four stages comprise our non-rapid eye movement (NREM) sleep, and the fifth stage is when rapid eye movement (REM) sleep occurs.

NREM sleep

Across this stage of sleep, we progress from being awake to sleeping deeply. During this process there is little muscle activity, and our eyes don't usually move; however, our muscles retain their ability to function.

REM sleep

During this final stage of sleep, we have bursts of rapid eye movements and this is the stage of sleep when most dreaming occurs. Our eyes are not constantly moving, but they do dart back and forth, and up and down. The reason for these eye movements is still a mystery. Although our eyes are moving rapidly, the muscles that move our bodies are paralysed while other important muscles, such as our heart and diaphragm, continue to function normally.

•••

Regardless of when you fall asleep, people tend to experience more NREM sleep in the earlier hours of the night and more REM sleep in the later hours of the night.

An expert in the field

Olivia Arezzolo

Olivia is Australia's leading sleep expert, speaker, author, coach and advisor. Her mission is to help individuals feel their best, inside and out, via sleep, and she has a profoundly unique articulation of sleep science.

According to Olivia's thorough research on sleep, evidence reported in *The Journal of Nursing Research* in 2019 indicates that 75 per cent of people who consume alcohol before bed wake too early and 69 per cent struggle to stay asleep. Many wake around 3 am with a chaotic stream of thoughts.

This is in part due to the REM rebound effect.[1] After alcohol's sedative effects have worn off, you have an exacerbated spike in awakening the hormone cortisol, to rebalance the nervous system. This often occurs around 3 am as there is a natural rise in cortisol around this time, due to the circadian rhythm[2]. Alcohol reduces REM sleep, and this sleep stage is more prevalent in the last third of the night, which may be the cause of 3 am, 4 am or 5 am waking. Sound familiar? These overnight interruptions limit sleep depth, resulting in less time spent in slow-wave (deep) and REM sleep, and more time in light sleep — and of course, more time awake. According to an article in the journal *Substance Abuse* in 2009, since sleep depth is as important as sleep length, alcohol consumption only contributes to the sleep debt cycle.

The consequences of not having enough good-quality sleep can include:

+ *Fatigue.* During sleep our bodies produce the human growth hormone, which is the key catalyst for muscle repair. In fact, research by the University of Chicago

---

[1] The REM rebound effect is the increase in frequency, depth and intensity of rapid-eye-movement (REM) sleep to compensate for sleep deprivation or significant stressors.

[2] Circadian rhythm is the natural cycle of physical, mental and behavioural changes that the body goes through in a 24-hour cycle. Circadian rhythms are mostly affected by light and darkness and are controlled by a small area in the middle of the brain.

(continued)

found that 70 per cent of the human growth hormone is produced in slow-wave sleep. So, if you're waking up fatigued and finding the simplest of tasks challenging, it's likely you haven't spent enough time in deep sleep and/or sleep altogether.

+ *Suppressed immune system.* As noted in a 2015 study by the University of California, you are over four times more likely to catch a cold if you sleep for six rather than seven hours at night. Yes — just one hour less escalates your risk of becoming unwell by around four times. This is in part due to the 70 per cent decline in immune agents, which usually detect and kill invading pathogens.

+ *Workplace errors.* Lack of sleep impairs your frontal lobe — the brain region responsible for decision making, judgement and time management. A 2016 sleep survey by Australia's Sleep Health Foundation found that 29 per cent of workplace errors can be directly attributed to fatigue. Yes — that's almost one in three. If that's you, please don't feel like there's something wrong with you. Your body is just trying to communicate that you need more sleep.

+ *Brain fog.* A 2018 study published in the journal *Proceedings of the National Academy of Science* found that for each night you don't sleep enough, your level of beta-amyloid (Aβ), a neurotoxin that contributes to brain fog, memory impairment and Alzheimer's disease increases by 5 per cent. This happens each night — let alone after weeks, months or years of insufficient sleep.

+ *Anxiety.* The University of Chicago found that just one night of insufficient sleep can see the stress hormone cortisol increase by 37 per cent. After two nights, it's 45 per cent. The consequences of this include an inability to switch off, feeling 'wired but tired' and mental rumination.

What's the good news?

Once you take alcohol out of your world, your body will be able to learn good sleep habits and eradicate the sleep debt cycle. Without alcohol, your natural circadian rhythm returns, and you begin to skip in step with the universe. You will be able to find better quality and quantity sleep, which will have a positive impact on almost every area of your life.

Alcohol and cancer

Alcohol is a toxin, so we know it increases the risk of certain cancers of the gastrointestinal system, oesophagus, stomach, liver, as well as breast cancer.
Dr Buddhi Lokuge, addiction expert, PhD, MD

In 2015 the Australian Institute of Health and Welfare estimated that around 4.5 per cent of all cancers are attributable to long-term, chronic use of alcohol each year in Australia.

In its Report on Carcinogens (5th edition), the National Toxicology Program of the US Department of Health and Human Services lists consumption of alcoholic beverages as a known human carcinogen. The American Society of Clinical Oncology (ASCO) advises that alcohol intake is an established risk factor for several cancers. Further to this, the American Cancer Society (ACS) 2020 guidelines advise complete avoidance of alcohol specifically for cancer prevention due to an increased cancer risk evidenced by alcohol consumption.

What is a carcinogen?

Carcinogens are substances that have the potential to cause cancer. There is overwhelming evidence to suggest that the more alcohol a person drinks on a regular basis over periods of time, the higher the chance of an alcohol-associated cancer developing. Not only that, but people who have no more than one drink per day have a moderately increased risk of some cancers, and based on National Cancer Institute data from 2009, an estimated 3.5 per cent of cancer deaths in the United States — approximately 19 500 deaths — were alcohol related.

According to the International Agency for Research on Cancer's GLOBOCAN, there are multiple ways alcohol consumption increases cancer risk in humans, namely:

- by breaking down the ethanol in alcohol to acetaldehyde, a toxic chemical and probable carcinogen

- by generating chemically reactive molecules, which can damage DNA proteins and lipids

- by impairing the body's ability to break down and absorb a variety of nutrients

- by increasing the levels of estrogen, a sex hormone linked to breast cancer risk.

Despite what you may have read on wellness websites, there is *no evidence* from studies in human populations to indicate any alcohol consumption provides protection against cancer.

Kathryn's story

Kathryn Elliott's relationship with alcohol started as a teenager in the 1980s, where she grew up in a normalised binge drinking culture (didn't we all?). Drinking in large amounts was considered a badge of honour and Kath, like many of us, spent most of her weekends drinking to excess. This continued into her 20s, 30s and 40s. Taking a significant break from drinking during her pregnancies and sometimes just to have a break for her health, Kath would always find herself back at the same spot — regretting the eventual blow-out night when she lost control.

In 2019, at age 46 and still binge drinking despite her desire to stop, Kath took some time away from alcohol and finally started to feel free from its relentless grip. But, as can happen in life, she was thrown a curveball. At the end of August 2019, Kath discovered a large lump in her right breast and two days later was diagnosed with locally advanced breast cancer, which rocked her to the core.

'As the shock of my breast cancer diagnosis started to settle, I found myself asking questions about my lifestyle, feeling uneasy about the role that alcohol had played and wondering whether this could have contributed to my diagnosis. I hadn't seen or heard much about the links between alcohol and breast cancer, so I decided to investigate myself. There were more than 100 studies that absolutely showed a direct link between alcohol consumption and increased breast cancer risk. I felt frustrated that I had never come across this information and wondered why there wasn't a more publicly visible health campaign about this issue, given breast cancer is the most diagnosed cancer in Australia affecting more than 20 000 people every year.'

Kathryn is a breast-cancer survivor and lives an alcohol-free lifestyle. She spends her days working as a specialist alcohol and binge drinking coach and advocating for better education on the links between alcohol and cancer, in particular breast cancer. Education is important when we are talking about alcohol, and although this information might seem heavy to digest, understanding the potential increased risks alcohol consumption exposes you to, can act as an excellent driver in shifting you towards choosing sobriety. A significant time away from alcohol will have many invisible benefits, one of which is a reduced risk of getting cancer.

Summing up ...

+ There is no safe amount of alcohol for human consumption.

+ Alcohol has no benefit to your body or your brain and can impact your sleep health negatively.

+ Alcohol, due to its effect on certain brain chemicals, can create an unhealthy cycle of drinking to feel good, then feeling bad and then drinking to feel good again.

+ Alcohol can lead to a long list of health issues; its impacts are physical and mental.

+ Alcohol is a sleep thief and can contribute significantly to sleep debt, which in turn has many knock-on negative impacts.

+ Alcohol is a carcinogen. It is cancer-causing in the human body and this is evidenced by scientific studies.

+ Despite the multi-faceted negative impacts of alcohol consumption on our brain, physical body and mental health, the good news is that by cutting alcohol out of the equation the many benefits for our body and brain are evident and previous damage that alcohol has caused can be reversed.

Now that you are aware of the impact alcohol can have on your brain, your body and your sleep, let's take a closer look at your relationship with alcohol and try to figure out why you drink so much and so often.

3 Assessing alcohol

'But why, Mum?'

A question my toddler asks me 100 times a day. About almost anything. *Why can't I fly a helicopter?* Because you are three. *Why can't I have a tractor?* Because there is nowhere to park it. *Why can't I have an ice-cream?* Because you just had one. I am trying my best to be the mum who doesn't return fire with a moderately moody, 'Because I said so'. I do my best to give my inquisitive threenager a toddler-appropriate explanation.

Here's a recent conversation from our evening walk around the block, during which we must go past the homewares shop with the tree of lights in the window display and walk past the payphone, which is now technically a freephone and really dates that Maroon 5 song about a payphone:

'Mum, can we call Dad from the phone box?'

'No darling.'

'Why?'

'Well, if the light is on, then the phone box is broken, and we can't make a call from a broken phone. Maybe it will be fixed tomorrow.'

Hands up who knows the light being on in the payphone box doesn't mean it's broken. Okay, so yes, this is a flat-out fib, but you do what works when you are in the parenting trenches, right? My point here is, I love all the questioning (most of the time) by my little one. So curious, all the time, about absolutely *everything*. And it has encouraged me to keep my curiosity on. Like we keep our manners on. There is a sweet innocence about always wanting to know why: why it must be, why it can't be different, why it is so. Why don't you know? Let's channel that inquisitive toddler who lives inside us all (or possibly with you). Now, before you yawn and skip to the next juicy chapter in the book, sobriety is a doing activity, and there will be some stop down moments throughout this chapter to help you identify and articulate your relationship with alcohol. The goal here is to define your relationship with alcohol so you can redefine it altogether.

Problematic drinking

So, your drinking behaviour hasn't exactly been like a scene from *The Hangover*, but you aren't exactly sober either. So what are the telltale signs that you might need to take a break from drinking and have a re-think about alcohol and its role in your life? When it comes to grey area drinking and binge drinking, it's not so clear. For some it's a slow burn and their relationship with alcohol can slowly become problematic. For others it's clear-cut denial that keeps them in the blame-shame endless cycle. Let's take a look at some signs of problematic drinking to help you identify your current relationship with alcohol.

Casey's story

Casey Davidson, a sobriety and life coach based in Seattle, Washington realised her drinking had become problematic by identifying some key behaviours for herself before going sober. Her high-flying corporate success had taken a toll and her drinking had become a daily habit.

'I had a few things leading up to my last drink that made me think at some point I was going to need to stop drinking eventually or soon... it was typical for me to just open and finish the whole bottle in a night and consider opening a second bottle. I didn't think it was unusual. I kind of woke up with a headache and a hangover every day and I would do the thing where I promised myself I would take a break to get in shape, pull myself together or whatever and then I would make it four days, and then think to myself, *Screw it. I need a bottle because today's been hard or good or my husband is away, or I'm bored.* So, then I'd go and buy a bottle of wine at night, and I would tell myself, 'Well if I do it every four days that's like two bottles a week. That's way better than nine bottles', which was the number of bottles I would drink when I was not trying to be good.'

Warning signs

There are many different signs your relationship with alcohol has run its course. Listed below are some obvious behaviours associated with grey area drinking, binge drinking and alcohol misuse. Acknowledging these behaviours, if they are present for you, will help you in clearly identifying your relationship with alcohol and guide you in understanding more about 'why' you drink alcohol. These aren't all the red flags, but if it makes you feel any better, by the time 2014 rolled around, I was doing a lot of this stuff without any idea they were clear indicators that I needed an alcohol re-frame. I felt normal. I felt okay. I thought I was kicking life in the pants, but when I took the time to assess my alcohol intake and its effect on me, I realised things were heading in a direction I was uncomfortable with.

This is an opportunity for you to have an honest assessment of your drinking habits and if you find yourself nodding along to this list like you would a Lizzo track, just know it's okay. This is part of the assessment process.

You'll find that some key statements in Casey Davidson's story are articulated and explained in the next section.

Eating is cheating

I need food! Some food-related warning signs are replacing food with alcohol, using meal times as an *excuse* to drink and ordering food to soak up your alcohol content rather than enjoying the simple pleasure of eating.

Oh, my head

I wake up with a headache and a hangover every day. We are not supposed to suffer through a headache caused by alcohol every day. The knock-on effects of a hangover can impact our sleep, nutrition, relationships and work ethic. A hangover a day does not help you work, rest and play.

I need a drink because...

I need a bottle because today's been hard. This is when you're unable to cope with life stuff, or get through a day, without feeling like you need a drink, or that a drink will take the edge off.

It's just the alcohol talking

Yes, it is, *or is it?* Check if your behaviour is becoming problematic or out of character. If your persona changes when you're drinking, you have an alter-ego when using alcohol. You become wild in the aisles or you don't remember having conversations when intoxicated.

Just one more drink/glass/bottle

It was typical for me to just open and finish a whole bottle in a night and consider opening a second bottle. If you find it difficult to have just one drink or if you're ordering a bottle of bubbles with a straw instead of a few glasses to share (guilty), you may have found yourself with more of a *stopping* problem than a drinking problem. This is still problematic. You might feel like you can't trust yourself around alcohol because you don't know when you'll stop.

I blacked out. I don't remember. What are you talking about?

If you've had a night out and you can't remember the next day, or if part of an evening or conversations are hazy, you've experienced a blackout. This is when alcohol starts messing with your memory and you don't know how you got home, who you said what to or why there is a purple wig on your lounge room floor! This reaction to over-consumption of alcohol is particularly dangerous.

I don't have a drinking problem, ya dumb cow

If someone has tried to discuss your drinking behaviour with you and you've been offended, defensive, aggressive or rude towards that person, this can indicate you are uncomfortable with your drinking behaviour and feel threatened when it is questioned. Your defensiveness is evidence of problematic drinking.

Well, Stacy* was way more drunk than I was

It's a warning sign when you always find a good excuse to drink by giving yourself invisible boundaries, such as 'I'm not as drunk as that person', or 'I'm not hurting anyone'. Simply, 'not hurting anyone' doesn't imply that no-one is hurt or the unhelpful 'that's way better than' self-talk is a clear indication your consumption needs to be questioned.

   * Stacy is a fictional person.

Porky pie

Another warning sign is when you downplay the number of drinks you have had, lie about your alcohol consumption, drink in secret, hide alcohol in your house or mask your alcohol consumption by drinking alone where no-one can hold you accountable.

Thinking about drinking

This is when you are constantly thinking about when you can have a drink, or when it will be appropriate to have a drink, such as 'It's my birthday so I'll sip Bacardi' (you know … like 50-cent); 'The kids are at my mum's for the weekend'; 'It's beer o'clock somewhere in the world' or if you walk into your friend's house and you go straight to the fridge to get a West Coast Cooler instead of a tub of hommus.

Broken promises

I promised myself I would take a break. But you can't stick to a limit you've given yourself around alcohol, or are breaking promises you've made to yourself about the number of drinks or the occasions you will or will not drink at.

I blew my finger off with a firework on the Millennial night. I have done some crazy things, but I have no shame. I was drunk and

I was heavily inebriated. I have left that in the past. I am not bringing my shame into my sobriety. That person does not represent the person who I am today.
Victoria Vanstone, alcohol-free living advocate

A friendly warning about the warning signs

This exercise is not to incite shame. It is to help you identify your relationship with alcohol as part of the wider process. The shame-blame cycle can be crippling. I know — I lived trapped in it for a long time. My encouragement for you is to show yourself compassion in this moment. Be kind to yourself with your self-talk. Take a breath, keep self-compassion at the top of your priority list as you read through the warning signs and try not to take on any guilt. What's done is done and when we know better, we do better.

Sobriety superpower: journalling

When it comes to identifying, accepting and changing your relationship with alcohol, journalling can be an excellent tool. Journalling helps to keep the brain active; it can improve our memory and comprehension skills, which may result in some improvement in cognitive function. Not only this, but journalling can also be a wonderful self-care tool, enabling better management of daily life stress. Journalling is an example of an expressive coping method: a wellness tool that can help people process their feelings, experiences and thoughts by writing them down. According to Krista K Fritson, Assistant Professor in the Department of Psychology at the University of Nebraska, writing down our thoughts is said to act as a form of release. Once the ideas swimming in your head and consuming your self-talk are written onto a page, they have less power. Studies show the emotional release from journalling lowers anxiety and stress and improves sleep. I was under the impression that a vodka, lime and soda would help me decompress from a hectic day. But I was mistaken. It turns out writing is much more beneficial.

Ever since I was a youngster coupling my primary school uniform with Reebok pumps, I have kept some form of writing practice. In year 5 I was awarded an A+++ for my written comprehension and reporting skills. Yeah, I know — I was a nerd. In the early 1990s, once a week our teacher would wheel across a fat-back TV, plug it into the wall at the front of the classroom and play an episode of *Behind the News* (*BTN*). This was my favourite time of the week, mainly because I knew I was so good at remembering and articulating the stories presented on *BTN* that I would get an A+++ for my report. I just loved the validation and so I practised writing from a young age — and I guess at some point I got good at it.

Later, in high school, as an awkward teenager who tried the perm trend and realised it wasn't for me, I kept a diary with its own code of how many sit-ups I had completed each day, which boy I had a crush on during the school term; and lots of teenage banter about the popular group at school (which I was not in), how much money I had saved towards my goal of buying my first pair of clogs (it was the '90s, remember) and what was happening between Kelly and Brandon on *Beverly Hills: 90210*.

In my 20s, journalling became commonplace, and the diary banter switched to monthly goals, savings plans, fitness challenges and what was going on between Ross and Rachel on *Friends*.

If your first thought is, 'but I'm not the writing type', that's okay. Not everyone is.

Here's your challenge!

Use this time of self-exploration to learn a new skill. Writing can be one of the new skills you learn and practise throughout this time in sobriety. If you are stuck as to where to start, don't worry. I will happily hold your non-dominant hand, as you'll have a pen in the other, and help you along the way. What would be great, just for now, is for you to be open to this idea. Much like juggling. You can only become a juggler if you start juggling. And then maybe one day you become a good juggler and run away with the circus! Or you might just whip it out at the odd birthday party. It's up to you. If writing is not your strong suit today, I am excited about what you are going to learn throughout this process. And if it is something you are familiar with or even an expert at, I am as excited for you to develop this practice further.

As I have mentioned, please keep an open mind, put aside everything you currently believe about yourself and come on the journey. Throughout this process there are written activities for you to complete, and if you are ever getting stuck, you can start with being grateful.

An attitude of gratitude

It is said that gratitude turns what we have into enough. Research by the Greater Good Science Center at UC Berkeley in 2021 suggests a practice of gratitude can have a positive effect on a person's mental health and can counteract negative thought patterns. A gratitude journal entry can simply be one thing you are grateful for, or it can be a longer piece of expressive writing. Let's take this journalling business and put it into practice.

Activity: gratitude journalling

Take out your journal and write down one thing you are grateful for. It may be a person, a memory, a feeling, a material item or a relationship — you might even write an essay. No pressure! Writing is an investment of your time. Trust me: I am writing a book! You might be wondering how you will have the time to both read this book and write details in your journal. One thing I discovered early on in sobriety is how much time you get back when you're not drinking. Remember

(continued)

all that time you used to drink alcohol, at the bar, on the couch with a nightcap? If you took an inventory of how much that is, my guess is that it would add up to be substantial. The time has always been there. You used it to drink in the past, but moving forward you can use it in so many new, empowering, beautiful and productive ways. Time is one of our greatest commodities and you're in control of how you spend your time. I understand you have responsibilities — a job, a business, a side hustle, an online store, children, ageing parents — but if you can see this as an opportunity to give something to yourself, what this process will unlock for you is so worth it. It might be a new thing to flesh out your feelings, and get whatever is in your head or your heart out on paper, but it's a key part of becoming acutely aware of your position and your feelings about alcohol. Just as we all have our own unique fingerprints, voice and way of tying a bin bag, we each have our own unique writing style. There is something profoundly intimate about expressing yourself in the written word.

Once you start, you'll find your flair.

First drinks to last drinks

I had my first drink when I was 15 years old. It was the end of a very successful end-of-year performance of *The Wiz*. I was absolutely easing on down the road to the after party. It was my first party. My parents had told me not to drink. Our teachers had told us not to drink. So, I drank. I drank rum straight out of the bottle. I had no idea what alcohol would do to my body. I hated the taste as I guzzled it down to fit in. I was hell bent on doing something I *wasn't allowed to do*. I passed out on the front lawn of the house where the party was being held before the music had even started. Thank God I was with friends, one of whom called her mum, who took me to her house and showered me in a bid to sober me up before she called my parents. There was talk of taking me to the hospital and although I couldn't articulate a sentence, I managed to convince my friend's mum not to. My mum was a nurse, you see, and the hospital was her place of work. My parents came and got me; it was a whole big dramatic scenario when my parents eventually collected me from my friend's house and drove me home. It was awful. I was so embarrassed. I was in so much trouble. This was the first, but not the last, time alcohol would see me throwing up, passing out and feeling humiliated.

In my early 20s, when I was wearing low-cut jeans, trying to force my way through the double denim trend and obsessed with *Will & Grace* — or, as I still call it, *Jack & Karen* — I would have a few drinks just for fun. Sure, some nights would be larger than others, resulting in a hazy recall of the end-of-night events, but despite the blurry end I had good mates and we looked after each other. Our weekend started on a Thursday night, and it was back-to-back nights of hanging out, dance floor shenanigans and the occasional messy bus trip home. I would always get to work, sometimes a little dusty, but *fine*: not great, not bad, just fine. It was *normal*. It was innocent, but it soon became a pattern of behaviour. Nothing seemingly went horribly wrong, but things did start to go pear shaped.

In 2004, after working at a radio station for a few years as a rookie producer, I landed my dream job on *MTV* as a VJ (TV host). Radio was fun, but I literally manifested my dream job. You see, I had written down in my journal when I was 15, around the time I was at that after party, that I wanted to be a VJ on *MTV*. A crazy dream for the late bloomer who didn't get boobs until year 11. Yet through a complicated roadmap of right time, wrong place, right place, wrong dress, rejection and winging it, I auditioned for a gig on *MTV* in 2004, and to my complete surprise, I was hired.

Suddenly I was *the girl from MTV* and living in my own manifested reality. I interviewed Blink 182 as my first assignment.

I was marketed as *the girl next door*: fun, smart, with just the right amount of sass. My life changed overnight. My on-camera chutzpah, my outgoing personality, my unique look (*MTV*'s words, not mine) were the talk of the town. It was amazing. Red carpets, business-class flights overseas, interviews with rock stars and pop stars, movie premieres and parties. And I drank as much alcohol as the next person. Very quickly my week became a busy hustle of events, openings, lunches, meetings, dress fittings, interviews, hair and makeup, and hosting TV shows.

I hit the ground running and it wasn't long before I felt an overwhelming sense of, 'How did this happen to me?' Along with the glamour of it, came the criticism about my personal style, and my eagerness to strike an air guitar pose in any photoshoot was quickly shut down. The executives' 'tweaks' came from a place of brand alignment, but I felt personally attacked. I started to feel very quickly that somehow this was all a big fluke, a mistake. I didn't fit in with the glamorous crowd of famous, beautiful people I was now circling around. I was great on TV. I was great at interviewing superstars and celebrities. I was calm, calculated and always well researched. Kanye West noted this after our chat about who he wrote the song 'Gold Digger' for originally. It wasn't Jamie Foxx, FYI. I was a hit. I had made it! But each day I woke up with compounded feelings of anxiety.

So, I drank.

I was wined and dined, shown endless bar tabs and backstage passes. There were limitless parties and endless amounts of alcohol being put in my glass, stashed in my bag and thrown down my throat. *It was normal.* A drink calmed my nerves before photographers shouted my name as I posed awkwardly in a barely-there dress and uncomfortable heels on a red carpet. I much preferred being on the other side of the divider, *asking* the questions, holding an *MTV*-branded microphone — my badge of honour. But somehow, I found myself straddling both sides of that red velvet rope like a rhythmic gymnast. The spotlight became my home, but it felt more like a microscope. I couldn't relax until I had a drink in my hand. Alcohol quickly became a comfort to me. It was weird. I guess this was the beginning of imposter syndrome, which only got deeper with each year I spent fronting the pop culture brand that every kid dreamed of being on. Counterbalancing the feelings of insecurity was alcohol. It was always there: at the door, in my glass, at the bar, as a nightcap. Alcohol became my companion. My trusted friend who would never let me down. Until eventually it did.

Now, I'm not blaming the music or TV industry for my alcohol dependence. There are many complex reasons as to how alcohol became the common thread in the fabric of my story. I'm just giving you some context. Working in a fast-paced VIP space, consumed by keeping up with everyone before *The Kardashians* were a household name and trying to stay relevant and edgy and represent a youth brand with the perfect mix of style and sass. It was a lot. The feedback I was receiving on my 'image', my popularity, my weight, my skin and down to the chip in my nail polish, was a lot. I felt over-managed, under-valued and insecure.

So, I drank.

Osher's story

I have known Osher Günsberg since he was Andrew G on Channel [V], one of the shiniest TV stars in Australia. Osher and I were on rival music TV platforms around the same era, and he, like me, had a problematic relationship with alcohol. His dates to Brisbane in the early 1990s.

'I learned how to drink in a cohort of people, and we weren't any more or less wild than the other people around us at the time, but you know, this is Brisbane drinking — it's

(continued)

essentially country drinking. I had a group of people that was essentially, "we're drinking...get your gumboots because this doesn't stop". You know, it's a good night if someone's vomiting through their nose. We called it the double dragon...that's what drinking meant. I didn't know that drinking could be anything else and so that's how it started.'

There's the bottle of champagne for a job well done, rooftop drinks on a Friday, an open bar at lunch for a good result, an open bar at lunch for a bad day. Then there's the off-site all-day meeting, the annual strategy session, tools-down tinnies, the on-site around the grounds and of course the end-of-year celebration. At home, it's the job of parenting children, managing your marriage or searching for your soul mate. Whether it's toddler tantrums or tinder dates, binge-watching TV or baking for the charity cake stall, a drink can be the one sweet moment of relief.

So, we drink.

Irene's story

Irene Falcone, a serial entrepreneur, found herself overwhelmed after the sale of her first hugely successful online business 'Nourished Life', admitting she turned to alcohol to cope with her identity crisis.

'I sold my entire soul when I sold my first business and so I went from running a company to no longer running a company and I just didn't know what to do with myself anymore...it was when I lost my sense of purpose that drinking became accessible and available to me because I simply did not know who I was any more, and I didn't know how to find her. And so, I drank my entire wine cellar.'

In one form or another, every person you encounter is looking to be seen and wanting to be heard. And do you know how I know this? Oprah told me. Okay, well, she has mentioned it a few times. 'I see you. I hear you. What you say matters to me' are the words Oprah Winfrey is often heard uttering when discussing the common human experience and need for validation. You see, Oprah Winfrey has interviewed slightly more people than I have in her decades-long media career, and has reflected on her time. Whether she interviewed a father of three, a celebrity, a divorcee, a widow, a popstar, a sports star, an inventor or otherwise, her guest would always ask, 'Was that okay?' Even Beyoncé!

For me, it was confusing.

Despite being seen on TV and heard on radio for most of my adult life, I didn't feel seen or heard. Isn't that wild? There was always a hole — a gap — and I understand now, it's because I was co-dependent on alcohol. Undercover drinking, binging on the weekends, doing my best to cope, knowing I wasn't. The acceptance and validation I needed, needed to come from myself. I had a lack of self-worth and emotional intelligence to process those big, out-of-place feelings. I was swept up in the glamour, the endless parties and the bottomless drinks. My ability to smash beers with the boys and down daiquiris with the girls quickly became part of my infectious charm.

Alexa's story

Action Alexa, a high-performance coach and mental health advocate, explains how she picked up a bottle of whiskey to cope with personal stress during a major family crisis.

'I was teased at school for being too skinny, so I went to the gym on a mission for muscles. I needed a safe place where

(continued)

I felt connected. It was there I developed the connection between physical strength and mental toughness. But after my mum's suicide attempt, my dad turned to the bottle. He became an alcoholic until he died of liver cirrhosis. The opposite of addiction isn't sobriety; its connection. I found my first sense of connection at the gym and my second sense of connection when I found my dad's whiskey bottle. During the week I would work out and feel great, but on the weekends, I was drinking myself into oblivion. And the saddest thing is, I didn't drink because I liked the taste of alcohol. I drank because I didn't like myself.'

Whether it's imposter syndrome, grief, guilt, loss, pain, pleasure, stress or shame.

You drink.

I understand.

Understanding your relationship with alcohol is a necessary part of this process, so let's unpack that, shall we?

Activity: why do you drink alcohol?

There are no right or wrong answers here, and the answers may be complex, even painful, to acknowledge — but they are important. My advice is to spend some time answering these questions honestly and be kind to yourself throughout this process. Remember this isn't a test; this is an exercise in self-reflection. If writing doesn't feel right for you at this moment, just having a time of self-reflection would be beneficial. Ask yourself these questions internally, or out loud. Of course,

I encourage you to write the answers down, but self-talk is always a great option when sorting through the big questions about your relationship with alcohol.

- Is there a certain feeling you are chasing or running away from?

- Are there particular people you drink around or hide your drinking from?

- How much alcohol do you drink at a time?

- When do you most often drink?

- How does alcohol make you feel at the start and at the end of the night?

- Do you feel alcohol is having a positive or negative impact in your life and in what areas?

Once you are done, close your journal and take yourself out for some fresh air.

Let's leave it here for now. Good job. You are allowed to give yourself the time and space necessary to address this complex topic. Take it steady and get some rest. You may feel emotional — that's completely okay. Feelings are there to be felt.

If alcohol was a person

For me to gain a truly honest assessment of my relationship with alcohol, I gave alcohol a persona and then wrote very candidly about my relationship with this 'person'. Somehow, giving alcohol an identity made it easier for me to assess and articulate my relationship status. Here's my personal alcohol assessment from 2014.

We hang out every afternoon, yet I have begun to dread hanging out with you. You are always there. Even when I promise myself I am going to stay away, I end up with you. In fact, I am angry at myself for continuing to give in to your charm. I wish I could tell you what I really think: that I want you to go away and leave me alone. But everywhere I go, every social situation, at the end of every long day, every weekend, there you are. Waiting for me. Enticing me. Seducing me. Even if I find myself bored, I seek you out, reluctantly. I have no other choice. I am drawn into your grip. I can't stop. I need to stop. But I don't know how. It's so confusing. You help me forget about my problems. You take away those feelings I am afraid of. You help me relax. You help me sleep. But then — oh then — the anxiety, the hangover, the regret, the feeling of failure, kicks me so hard it hurts.

At first, we hung out as fun, but now I don't know how to function without you. How did this happen? Am I co-dependent? Am I going insane? You have an undeniable grip on me that I can't seem to escape. The very thought of trying to navigate my life without you seems impossible. I can't socialise without you. I can't get through an afternoon without you. I say I won't, then I do. I start and can't stop with you. No-one knows. It's my secret shame and I can't continue. This must end. But how?

I'm exhausted. I don't know who I have become or who I am without you. I am stuck. I hate how you make me feel, what you make me do. Things need to change between us.

When I conducted a self-assessment on my relationship with alcohol, I was able to get some real perspective on what my relationship with alcohol looked like. It was a hard reality check. If I had written the above about a person, you would be thinking, 'Maz, that person is toxic. That person doesn't care for, love or value you. You need to end that relationship.' And you'd be spot on. From the very raw realisation I was in a terribly toxic relationship with alcohol, I was better able to assess *why* I used alcohol and why I used so much of it, so often. With some time to reflect, I started to see the level of people pleasing I had self-assigned had left me with zero capacity to sustain myself. I overlooked my own needs in favour of making everyone like me. I was oversensitive, under a microscope and exhausted. My coping strategy of choice was a mix of adrenaline and alcohol. It kept my head above water, just barely, for an entire decade.

I have come to understand I suffered greatly from a fear of success way more crippling for me personally than any fear of failure. I have failed so many times and built grit and resilience through those moments. I have always looked at failure as the steppingstone to success. But success is a whole different ballgame. With failure you can calculate where things went wrong; you can correct the course, dust yourself off and try again. You can apply the lesson, keep calm and carry on. Success? I had no idea how to manage success and by this point, I had a great deal of it to deal with.

So, I drank.

It is a misconception to presume you must be falling-down drunk and hit absolute rock bottom to address your relationship with alcohol. Sure, I was drinking a lot more than is recommended, but I had my career, my face on billboards, my dream job. Having my outside life so together made it more difficult to understand my complex relationship with alcohol. My success was skewing my perception, but our perception is reality. Sobriety and shame, unfortunately, seem to go hand in hand. Ultimately, though, you are on a personal quest to answer the question, 'Am I okay with my relationship with alcohol?' It turns out I was categorically not okay with mine, so I did something about it.

> **It is a misconception to presume you must be falling-down drunk and hit absolute rock bottom to address your relationship with alcohol.**

I've come to view alcohol as a form of plutonium. It's nuclear for me. It's quite loaded, it's powerful, it radiates poison and if I put it in me, yeah, I am going to expire. It's very toxic for me, so it's off limits.
Yumi Stynes — media personality, sober since 2014

Activity: assessing your relationship with alcohol

Here are some questions you can ask yourself to dig a little deeper and find a way to articulate your relationship with alcohol. This is about how alcohol is impacting your life. This process is key in defining your current relationship with alcohol. Without a definition, there is no redefinition. This may take some journalling, counselling, a conversation and a bit of time. Sit with the questions and see what you come up with. (There are no incorrect answers. This is not a quiz!) Please write in your journal. There is no word count, there are no rules. This is your story and your relationship status. Remember, no-one needs to read this, and please be honest with yourself.

Write down what your relationship with alcohol is currently like. Explain your relationship with alcohol as if alcohol were personified, as if it were a relationship with a person, remembering that the person in this story is alcohol.

+ When do you and alcohol spend time together?

+ How often do you and alcohol spend time together?

+ Is alcohol around even when you don't want it to be?

+ Do you have feelings of guilt after you have spent time with alcohol?

+ How does alcohol make you feel?

+ How do you feel without alcohol?

+ Is alcohol having an impact on your other relationships or your work?

+ Is alcohol impacting your health?

When I was sober curious back in 2014, there weren't a lot of sober curious websites, podcasts, pamphlets, books or hashtags. I just googled 'Am I an alcoholic?' This did not prove to be helpful at the time. The term 'alcoholic' is tired, misleading and conjures up old-fashioned connotations. The term 'alcoholic' and the question of whether I was one didn't lead me any closer to being able to articulate what my relationship with alcohol was. From what I googled, I didn't think I was an alcoholic, but I knew I wasn't sober or at all comfortable with my relationship with alcohol. I hope the activity you just completed is a much more empowering way to assess where you and alcohol are at.

The impact of alcohol

Alcohol doesn't help you relax; it slows your brain, so you temporarily stop caring. That's not the same. Let me tell you a bit about my grey area/binge drinking, or alcohol misuse/overuse (or whatever you want to call it).

It all started to unravel when I was hosting *The Dan & Maz Show*, a national radio show broadcast across Australia from 4 pm to 6 pm weekdays. In fact, I still have people tell me that they miss the 'Dan & Maz magic' — it was a radio show that could have become one for the history books, but an unfortunate combination of mismanaged expectations, radio politics and, let's face it, flat out BS, shattered that dream at the end of 2015. Interestingly, this coincided with my first year of sobriety.

By 2014 alcohol had crept into my daily life. At all the work events I hosted or attended, I found myself in rooms where I felt equally as out of place as I was important. Drinking just wasn't questioned. I could swan around a room of celebrities and drink champagne until the sun came up: it was *my job*. I was the former host of *MTV*'s flagship show *Total Request Live (TRL)*, for goodness sake! And now I was on national radio. I was always safe, street-smart. I went to the gym and did spin classes at 6 am, so I was usually home by midnight — unless I wasn't. The gym did offer me a good excuse to get out of a super big night, though, and anyway, things were manageable. I was handling it. On the home front, if I wasn't going out, I would drink wine and make dinner and drink more wine with dinner. It helped me sleep, although it didn't help me remember the storyline of *How I Met Your Mother*, which I rewatched in early sobriety to finally understand how Ted Mosby met his wife!

Looking back now, I can see how it slowly got more of a grip as I lost touch with my true self and sought out other people's opinions of me. I can't put my finger on exactly when the shift occurred, but at some point, *I started drinking to cope*. My media career made drinking so easy and not drinking impossible. There was always someone who wanted to catch up for drinks, a place to go out for drinks or an event to get a drink at after we had been drinking. More and more occasions in my calendar involved alcohol: everything from a baby shower to backstage.

Blair's story

Blair Sharp is a mum of one from Minnesota, USA, now known as The Sobriety Activist. She remembers precisely this moment unfolding at her home in 2019, which led to her last drink.

'I had bought a couple of bottles of wine that night and of course I had drunk both plus whatever else was in the house. This was quite normal for me at that time. Except that night I happened to trip over the baby gate and drop my wine glass on the floor. It shattered, but again this wasn't out of the ordinary for me. I would fall a lot, I would break things, I was always losing things and it wasn't weird that I would have hurt myself. My husband came home as I was cleaning up the wine glass, and the next morning he told me that I could no longer drink alone with my son in the house: it just wasn't safe because we didn't know what would happen. And that was it. I was done with drinking.'

Some of the physical impacts of my alcohol consumption, aside from many hangovers, night sweats and time spent on the bathroom floor, included bruises on my legs from falling over in heels, and on one occasion scaling a paddock fence at a winery (classy, I know), a twisted knee, a sprained ankle, a stiff neck, ripped jeans (the paddock fence again), grazed knees from a running incident (heels, again), a lost voice and a black eye from misjudging an elevator door. Other impacts my alcohol consumption included were lost property: several wallets, a few winter coats, a couple of wigs, front door keys, a top hat, a handbag (at a nightclub), an entire suitcase (left in the back of a taxi with a brand-new hair straightener in it), two phones (to be fair, one was stolen from my handbag at a different nightclub), hundreds of dollars in cash from over-tipping and the heel of a high heel. Yes, I managed to break a high heel and stay out past the time Cinderella turned into a pumpkin.

I was trapped in a vicious and destructive cycle. I desperately wanted to calm my farm on the booze front, but I had no clue where to start. I would tap into Dry July and get through a month without alcohol to prove I didn't have a problem, only to have a very 'wet August'. At the time, I thought if I can stop for a month, then I am okay, right? Wrong. By 2014, with the ink still wet on my national drive show contract, I inherited an overwhelming feeling: imposter syndrome. I didn't feel talented enough to get the job, even though I got the job! Drinking was my coping mechanism to manage the stress I was under. I'd relocated to three different cities in three years and navigated a divorce at age 30. The compounded grief of some very real and big events led me to reach for the bottle more in 2014 than I had in the past and pushed down those big feelings further. So, there it is. It was my inability to process some big disappointments and stressors in my life that led me to lean towards alcohol more and more. The mental health impacts of my alcohol consumption didn't present clearly at the time; however, on reflection my levels of social anxiety were heightened. I had night terrors some evenings, broken sleep, an overactive imagination where I would catastrophise dramatic situations, a fear of missing out, a fear of losing my job, memory loss and feelings of loneliness. The relational impacts of my alcohol consumption led to me lying about my consumption of alcohol, feelings of shame and pretending I was okay. When I wasn't. I was lonely. I was unable to be honest with myself or my friends about what was really going on for me, behind the scenes, off-air, in the side of stage wings. I was guarded. I had built a cage around myself to protect a secret way of coping with life that wasn't working anymore. At the time, thoughts of inferiority were silenced with sips of wine. The shame was shoved down with shots. I drank myself numb because I didn't know how to process the emotions that came with the pressure. Nobody explained to me that my inner drive to be successful, to be seen and heard, would be riddled with doubt. At some point alcohol became my closest friend, the ultimate mask, and I wore it well.

Activity: how alcohol impacts you

Here are some questions about the impacts of alcohol on you. Answer them honestly. Remember, the notes you write in your journal are just for you. It's an important way to organise your thoughts and feelings around the dense topic of your relationship with alcohol. So be honest. Don't hold back. This is about getting to the core truth of your situation so we can work together in turning it around.

+ Is your relationship with alcohol having any negative impact on your physical health and wellbeing?

+ On your mood and mental health?

+ On your relationships?

+ On your work life, social life or other areas?

+ What specifically are those negative impacts?

The catalyst (spoiler alert: someone dies)

I raced from *The Dan & Maz Show* to my hair appointment. I was flustered navigating Melbourne traffic on a Friday afternoon, not yet used to the trams and traffic of a city I'd called home just shy of a year. I was super excited about finally getting my hair done at a very fancy, sought-after salon. I was already on a high from doing a Friday afternoon show, the most fun show of the week, a 'Friday fun one' and with a new 'do on the horizon'. I was getting my hair coloured purple: so chic, so in like Flynn — and nothing could dampen my mood. I swung open the salon door and gave my name to the beautiful man at the front desk. It was like being greeted by a Ken-doll. I was ushered to wait on a comfortable leather couch by the window with 'Hairdresser of the Year' plastered across it. Subtle. I sipped on a champagne. I always had a champers (or two) at the salon, darling, and passed the time scanning the pile of posh fashion magazines on the coffee table.

My phone rang.

It was odd for my phone to ring on a Friday evening, especially when I saw it was Entertainment Management, the landline of my management team based in Sydney. I'd been with Mark Byrne Management for seven years and continued as a client when the business transitioned into Entertainment Management headed up by the most talented talent manager, Mark Andrew Byrne. We had dinner booked in Melbourne for the following week.

Mark was more than a manager. He was a dear friend and someone who believed in me, someone with whom I trusted my dreams. From the moment I met Mark, a light went on inside me, a little piece that lit up like never before — something truly special. And I feel like a little bit of him lit up when he met me too. We shared many conversations about purpose and philosophy, about an industry we hated and loved, happiness and authenticity. I trusted Mark. He always went with his gut, encouraging me to decline opportunities that didn't feel right, rather than take the pay cheque. He taught me that when you take the high road, the view is always better, and although the road may be longer, you appreciate it so much more. Mark is why I moved to Adelaide in 2011 to host my first breakfast radio show. He told me it felt right, and I agreed, even though it didn't make logical sense at the time. We went with our guts, and we were right. Two years later, I was poached by another radio network and returned to Sydney as half of a fully backed radio duo, *The Dan & Maz Show*, and just a year after that I was hosting the *National Drive Show* out of Melbourne and getting my hair done at a super fancy salon. We were a dream team. Mark took big risks. He was fearless and calculated. He always encouraged me to do everything with grace and style. He invested in my abilities and taught me not just to dream crazy but to do the very thing I was afraid of. Because, after all, we humans are surprising creatures, and there is so much more in us than we sometimes dare to believe.

'Who else is going to be Maz Compton?' he would say.

Mark was a busy guy, and he would usually call from his mobile while in a huge rush to be somewhere important and usually running late, so it was a little strange for the landline number to come up, but I just figured it was most likely one of the team checking in to confirm dinner for next week, so I answered…

I almost sang my cheerful greeting as I stepped outside the noisy salon.

'Hello and to what do I owe the pleasure?'

Silence

'Hello? He-llo?'

Silence

'Hi Maz, It's David.'

David, a lovely British chap who I always had a laugh with on the phone, was my day-to-day contact at the business and oversaw my schedule. He made sure I knew where I needed to be and had all the information I needed to have. I like to think I was one of David's favourite clients and I had hoped this was a social call, but it wasn't.

'Maz, I'm so sorry to tell you this. I don't know what to say. Mark has died.'

Silence.

Shock.

Confusion.

And the intense feeling of the air being sucked from my lungs...

More silence.

I felt the colour drain from my face as I leaned against the window with Hairdresser of the Year plastered on it and slid down to the ground.

Anguish.

Anguish goes for your bones. It's more than sadness, despair and grief. I stared somewhere. Not into the salon, not out to the street. Just somewhere. I didn't hear much more of what David said in the following moments. I could feel my heart racing and my ears ringing.

The whole world completely stopped. I was frozen. I felt numb.

'Maz, are you there? Maz, I'm so sorry.'

David proceeded to tell me that Mark had died of a heart attack and was found earlier that day unresponsive at home in his kitchen. He was 45. He was dead. I was beyond devastated. I don't remember what I said to David, but he asked if I needed someone to come and get me, knowing that I was living away from my family. But I said I would call a friend. I hung up the phone and went back into the salon. I didn't cancel my appointment. I got my hair coloured purple. It's strange what you do when you're in shock. I watched call after call come to my phone and I let them ring out on silent. I could not believe what had happened. I pushed it out of my mind and carried on a semi-normal conversation with my colourist about stuff you talk to your colourist about: boys, Botox and Brangelina (it was 2014, remember, so this was a hot topic at the time). After my hair appointment I got into my car and I called my mum and told her the news. Then I called my boyfriend and told him too. All I could say was, 'Mark's died. I don't understand.' I was in shock.

I didn't cry for a few hours. It was when I spoke to a friend, Natalie, who was very close to Mark that I finally switched from disbelief to despair and the tears came in floods. When I got home to my apartment with my newly coloured hair, I called another friend, Tim, whom I had met through Mark. He stayed on the phone with me for a very long time and talked me through one of the roughest and loneliest nights of my life. I drank red wine.

Thank you, Tim. You were a true brother to me in my moment of devastation. You helped me be strong enough to carry through the pain and to accept the Mark-shaped hole in my heart.

Everything changed for me after Mark died. I started to look at my life from a very different perspective. I thought a lot about legacy. Did I just want to be another talking head on radio, filling the space with senseless banter, or did I want to make a difference in people's lives? What did I stand for? Who did I want to become? How could I make Mark proud? What did Mark see in me? Where could I find that? Why was I drinking so much?

Mark took a chance on me. He believed in me, dreamed my dreams with me and facilitated my career with such precision. Mark had created a beautiful family of misfits, and now we were orphans. I lost my friend, my confidante and my shepherd all at once, and my heart was broken. The days after Mark's death are a blur. I tried my best not to lose it, but it felt like I was never going to run out of tears. I wept for days and I drank a lot of wine. Then, three weeks after

Mark died, I was offered the job hosting the *Sydney Breakfast Show*. This was the job Mark had believed we could work towards seven years earlier. This was his grand plan manifesting in front of my own eyes, yet I couldn't share it with him. Mark encouraged me to work hard, hone my craft, do the time and learn the skills, and the rest would come. And it did. It was bittersweet accepting the job he and I had worked so hard for, without him there. As I accepted the job, I also came to realise I wasn't coping. I googled, 'Am I an alcoholic?' and was left with more questions, so I called Beyond Blue and had a long discussion with Susan.

The last time I saw Mark, I was his plus one to the opening of *The Lion King*. He was running late, as always, and we both cried during the show. With tears streaming down our faces, we managed to have a laugh about our obvious Daddy issues. It was a perfect final moment to share with him, and that's the circle of life.

Summing up ...

+ There are many red flags when it comes to identifying our relationship with alcohol. Acknowledging problematic drinking behaviour in your own life is a good first step towards sobriety.

+ Feelings of guilt can arise when assessing your drinking behaviour. Try not to engage with guilt, but acknowledge you are on a path to betterment.

+ Journalling is a sobriety superpower. There are many benefits to journalling about your feelings and this will help you define and redefine your relationship with alcohol.

+ Part of the process of identifying your relationship with alcohol includes asking yourself a lot of curly questions. Try to be honest with yourself about the answers.

(continued)

- A practice of gratitude can help to refocus your attention onto one positive thing.

- Defining why you drink alcohol and articulating your personal relationship with alcohol are keys for the foundation of your sobriety.

- Assessing your relationship with alcohol will help with the acceptance that you want it to change.

- A catalyst for change can come at any moment, but you can also just choose sobriety. Remember, you don't have to hit a rock-bottom moment to reassess your relationship with alcohol.

Now that you know all about alcohol and have made some headway on defining your current relationship with alcohol, let's talk about sobriety.

Part II

Sober curiosity

In part I we investigated the case for why alcohol is the problem. We looked at the various impacts alcohol can have on our brains, bodies, relationships and otherwise. You were presented with the challenge of articulating your current relationship with alcohol, and you have been able to identify some significant truths about alcohol, its role in your life and why you want to take a break.

So, what about this sobriety thing?

It turns out, sobriety works. Let's unpack exactly what sobriety is and start exploring how it's going to work for you. This is about pinpointing why you want to give sobriety a go and will equip you with clear steps and important tools you can use to navigate sobriety successfully — it will be your personal Sober Toolkit. Here is where the work begins, my friend. This is about creating awareness, setting an intention around your habits, understanding yourself and forming new behaviours.

I echo my encouragement here. Please keep an open mind, be honest and kind with yourself, and complete the activities — they will provide you with a solid foundation for sobriety and are an important part of this process. Let's begin with some sobering thoughts about sobriety and what to look out for as you navigate this season:

- Sobriety is a one-moment-at-a-time *process*.

- Sobriety is not a one-size-fits-all solution; there is no silver bullet or magic pill. This is a *learning journey*.

- Not drinking at all can sometimes be *easier than trying to moderate* and failing, so if you've been trying to moderate and are failing at it, this is reassuring.

- Sobriety isn't a quick fix for life's struggles, but it will give you a *clear head* and the emotional capacity to choose how to better navigate the tough life stuff.

- Some people simply won't understand why you are choosing sobriety, and that's okay. *They don't need to.*

- You will likely need support. Speak up and *ask for help*. Counselling, an online community or a good mate can help you through testing times.

- Prepare to *get comfortable with being uncomfortable*. This is where we grow.

- *Stay curious* babe and keep asking questions.

Gearing up for some time away from alcohol can feel overwhelming, but let's break it down into bite-sized chunks, shall we? Since you won't be drinking for the next few weeks, you will probably feel a bit out of sorts thinking about how much time you will have on your hands. This may feel uncomfortable at first, but it does become like your favourite pair of tracksuit pants — you know, super comfortable and breathable in the right places. There are no hard and fast rules for how to walk through this season, but seeing as I have danced this dance, let me show you around. I will help you pinpoint some key things to help you safeguard your sobriety. Find the sobriety tools that will work for you and apply those.

I've built a life in sobriety that I could never have imagined when I was drinking. I drank everything away. All the decisions I made when I drank led me to make financial and relationship decisions that ended up just wreckage for everybody involved, but what I have built since then, the rebuild, is only possible because I don't drink and my life is enormous and wonderful because I am sober.
Osher Günsberg — TV and podcast host, sober since 2010

4 Sobriety is the solution

Alcohol is the thread of the fabric of our society. It's entwined in how we engage socially. And when it's not working for you, it can feel suffocating — and it can feel impossible to escape from it. I understand this struggle so deeply because I wrestled with this for years. Wanting to get away from alcohol, yet there it was at every turn of the social diary. This for you right now might seem like a mountain too high to conquer. But I assure you, it's totally doable. Think about what alcohol promises and understand it is sobriety that delivers on those promises.

Memories of alcohol

When the alcohol I had been consuming almost every day of my adult life had finally drained out of my system, it felt like the creativity exploded in my head. My brain is wired in a particular way, as is yours, and from my limited knowledge about neuroscience, our brains can rewire. We can change our brains, and that's what you are edging towards. In my first month away from booze, I experienced a very profound paradigm shift in my creativity. It felt like suddenly there was a bright and electric buzz in my brain space. It didn't happen in the first week, but at some point during my sobriety plan, something clicked. A light switched on in my head. The fog cleared. The haze lifted. I felt like I could breathe deeper, sleep better. I was more patient and calmer, and I wasn't trying to be — I just was. This may not be the exact same for you, but I do hope you get to have your 'aha' moment when you realise this is worth it! I hope you find your switch too.

> *I drank for happiness and became unhappy. I drank for joy and became miserable. I drank for sociability and became argumentative. I drank for sophistication and became obnoxious. I drank for friendship and made enemies. I drank for sleep and woke up tired. I drank for strength and felt weak. I drank for relaxation and got the shakes. I drank for courage and became afraid. I drank for confidence and became doubtful. I drank to make conversation easier and slurred my speech. I drank to feel heavenly and ended up feeling like hell.*
> **Author Unknown**

The write decision

A big part of my early sobriety was documented in a journal. This has been stored safely in a box with my many copies of various Oprah biographies, unofficial and otherwise, Maya Angelou memoirs and Brené Brown's body of work. They are in a box because when I minimised, I got rid of my bookshelf and switched to audio books. The books I had read, I gave away as gifts and the ones I couldn't part with, I keep in a box in a cupboard, and that's where my journals are too. I mentioned in part I that I have mostly kept a writing practice of sorts and I found writing in a journal each day of my first month away from alcohol helped to keep me accountable and to process what was going on for me. Some days I wrote lots; other days little. And there were a few days when I didn't feel like writing, so I wrote about that.

A study by the Department of Linguistics at the University of Victoria noted writing is a part of the process and skill of language learning. It has a direct association with intelligence. Yes, writing increases your intelligence, smarty pants. See, it is a superpower and one you can totally engage during your early sobriety, so keep writing in your journal. You have already created a great starting point for your sobriety by identifying your relationship with alcohol and now we can build on this as we articulate your intention for this season of sobriety. Your journal, as you continue to add to it, will serve as a beautiful way to reflect on this process of self-learning, and as you find pockets of time and revelations present themselves, I hope you keep note of this life-changing time. During this season of sobriety, don't leave home without it. I'm sure that's a tagline for a product of some sort, but I can't quite put my finger on it. Anyway, journalling. It's priceless.

Our habits... and rabbits

Let's take a bit of a look at our habits and how we can hack them. And, for the record, it takes longer than 21 days to break a habit, but when you get to day 21 of any habit-formation process, it is significant. You have moved further towards the goal of creating effective change within yourself and the new habit is beginning to become more natural. So, what exactly is a habit and how do we change them?

What is a habit?

A habit is a settled tendency, a usual manner of behaviour. The Merriam-Webster dictionary calls it 'an acquired mode of behavior that has become nearly or completely involuntary'. In your case — as was mine — drinking. Another way to define a habit is as something that you do often and regularly, sometimes without knowing that you are doing it. Case in point. Now let's apply this definition to your drinking behaviour, and if you are like I was, drinking has most certainly become a regular, sometimes involuntary, habit. Now habits can be good *and* bad, but for the moment let's not moralise drinking. Let's just agree that your drinking behaviour has become a habit. Now that you can identify your drinking as a habit, we can unpack what that means and how you can change it. Awareness is the basis for learning new habits, but also for letting go of habits that don't serve us. We all want to believe it's our Instagram followers, our jobs, that charitable side hustle, those kids we're raising, our bank balance or snowboarding skills that define our character. But

Our habits become our character.

it's not any of those things. No, not even your ability to jump on the latest Tik Tok trend. What defines us, is our habits! *Our habits become our character.*

What makes a habit?

Psychology Today describes habit formation as the process by which new behaviours become automatic. If you instinctively reach for a coffee the moment you wake up in the morning, you have a habit. By the same token, if you pour yourself a glass of wine when you walk in the door after work, you've got yourself into a habit. Old habits are hard to break and new habits are hard to form because the behavioural patterns we repeat most often are literally etched into our neural pathways. The good news is, through repetition it's possible to form — and maintain — new habits. Understanding how our brains work can help us in the habit department. It is possible to hack into the system of our own minds to create new habits. This might sound a bit *Matrix*-y, but think of it as a ninja mind trick on yourself. Let's hear from a legit brain scientist about the neural pathways in our brains and how we can rewire them.

An expert in the field

Dr Ineka Whiteman

Neuroscientist Dr Ineka Whiteman explains how we can rewire the neural pathways in our brains.

As we saw in chapter 2, the brain is a highly dynamic organ, capable of changing and reorganising its neural networks in response to different input. Known as neuroplasticity, through our own conscious choices — whether we choose to have or to stop having a particular thought process — we have the ability to change the way our brain is wired, at the cellular level. The mind and our thoughts are such powerful tools, they enable us to perform a sort of 'micro-neurosurgery' on our own neural pathways, simply by choosing to think (or not think) in certain ways.

In terms of alcohol consumption, we also saw in chapter 2 that over time, it takes an individual ever more alcohol to feel good, which leads our drinking behaviour to progress from being relatively controlled and seemingly harmless, to us forming drinking habits, and eventually becoming dependent — where we go to extreme measures to ensure we get that feel good kick from drinking (usually excessive amounts) at the end of each day.

So how do habits form in the first place? If we can understand some of the 'nuts and bolts' of what happens to the brain as habits form, then I believe it empowers us as individuals with the tools we need to overcome those habits or — even better — to stop them forming and taking hold over our lives in the first place.

Habits so often begin with a thought. Just a single thought. It is said that the average adult has up to *70 000 thoughts each and every day*. That's *a lot* of thinking! If we tend to have the same kinds of thoughts over and over, and we put those thoughts into action over and over, we begin to wire stronger and stronger connections in our neural pathways. Eventually those thought processes become so strongly entrenched in our circuitry, that the associated behaviours become a habit. By definition, a habit is 'something that you do often and regularly, sometimes without knowing that you are doing it.' Another way of describing this is like being on 'autopilot'. Here's an everyday example. If you drive a car, chances are you have a familiar route you drive every day, to work, or the gym, or school drop off.

(*continued*)

When we first start driving this route, it takes a lot of conscious thinking, as our neural connections are just starting to form. Over time, thinking about the route as we're taking it and the actions of driving the same directions over and over become so strongly wired into our brains, that they eventually become a habit, and we don't even consciously think about the drive to work or school anymore — we drive on autopilot.

The same can be said of how drinking habits form. It might start with just one harmless thought. For example, 'It's been a tough day at work. I feel like a nice cold beer. When I get home this afternoon, I'm going to crack one. I deserve it.' If this thought leads to that action — the drinking of the beer, and the warm fuzzy pleasure sensation we get when we do this — the same thoughts and same actions over and over eventually become our habit. Our go-to every day after work, without us even giving it conscious thought. We walk in, put our keys down and go to the fridge for a beer.

If you're finding yourself sliding into this kind of drinking habit, or maybe you feel like you've already slipped off that cliff into the abyss, there is hope! No matter where you are on your sobriety journey, the first step to quitting alcohol is *believing that you can*. Because *you can*. You have the tools and equipment at hand, at this very moment, to put into action the changes you want to make. And it begins with the mind. A single thought, in fact. '*I can do this.*' Read that again.

Your brain doesn't control you and your habits. It's the other way around. You have the choice to unwire and rewire new habits into your brain, by changing the way you think. If we choose to stop having a particular thought, if we pull ourselves up each time we slip back to the old thought patterns then our brains will, over time, rewire the neural pathways.

It's literally mind over matter — brain matter, in this case!

Activity: becoming aware of your habits

Let's flesh this out in your journal. Spend some time thinking about each circumstance that comes up for you that leads you to reach for a drink. List them all down: every moment, every environment, every time. Do this without judgement. By creating awareness around the situations that have become habitual for you to consume alcohol, you can eventually rewire the neural pathways. For example, my list in 2014 looked a bit like this:

+ After-work drinks on the rooftop
+ Pre-event drinks while getting ready at home
+ Quiet night in with a movie and a bottle of red
+ Post-workout Savvy B to relax
+ Nightcap after a night out
+ Drinks at a party
+ Lunchtime beers on a weekend
+ I'm bored
+ I'm tired
+ I'm alone
+ I'm so busy
+ I'm excited
+ I'm with friends
+ I feel stressed
+ I need to sleep.

I understand this activity will be more challenging for some than others, but here is my encouragement: please keep an open mind, and go there. Go there with your honest self and

(continued)

do your very best to try and understand how drinking became your go-to habit. For some it is simply that you weren't taught any other coping skills for life, societal engagement, or ups and downs, so drinking became the one tool in your toolkit that you could apply to any given situation: *drinking is the multi-tool of coping*. The beautiful thing about this process is that once you know better, you can do better. I did.

Rabbits

Well, rabbits are cute!

Summing up ...

+ Alcohol is the problem, and sobriety is your solution.

+ A life without alcohol is better for your brain.

+ Journalling is a sobriety superpower and there is evidence to suggest it can increase your intelligence. Get writing and keep writing.

+ The process of sobriety is about creating new and healthier habits. Habit formation is a neural system that can be hacked. The wonderful thing about our brain is we can rewire it to form better habits.

+ Alcohol use keeps us in a position of only coping with the big life stuff and sobriety allows you the brain power and emotional intelligence to deal with the big life stuff. The big life stuff doesn't stop when you decide to stop drinking, but you give yourself the best opportunity to navigate life's ups and down with self-care and compassion, wisdom and authenticity.

Now that you know a bit about sobriety and what is has to offer, let's look at some practical ways sobriety can help you embrace your best self.

5 Sobriety is a superpower

Let's peek behind the curtain of sobriety and dig into some real-life measures of how impactful sobriety can be. In this chapter we explore some practical ideas about what sobriety will bring to your life and the positive impact it can have in many areas. In my experience, sobriety is a superpower: it is the unspoken secret to how to be your best self. It is your greatest asset, your biggest truth, your best chance at living a meaningful life filled with purpose. Sobriety will explode your life in the best way possible. And I'm not the only one who can attest to this.

> *After I had stopped drinking for a little bit, my life just got so much better. My anxiety went down, I felt better physically, and I even ran a 10 k fun run. My house was calmer and more peaceful. I decided to do a full six-month alcohol-free stint. My husband was shocked. We were going on vacation to Italy and Croatia and I was the girl who loved red wine! But once I knew how good things were for me and my family, I kind of went, 'You know what, I'm done with drinking for good.'*
> **Casey Davidson — sobriety coach**

Sobriety is self-care

When I stopped drinking, at first I did it just for the month of January 2015. After having that season of time processing Mark's death, and doing some self-assessment, I knew I wanted to take some time away. Honestly, I thought I was going to be *so bored*. I had no idea how I was going to get through an entire weekend without a drink. But I took to the experiment with an open mind, as you are doing, to see how *not drinking* looked on me, to see who I could find looking back at me in the mirror. What I uncovered was far beyond any of my expectations. What I realised is that sobriety is the definition of self-care.

Self-care is not self-indulgence or being selfish. Self-care means actively taking care of yourself so that you can be healthy, you can be well, you can do your job, you can help and care for others and you can do all the things you need to and want to accomplish in a day. You can liken self-care to the safety instructions on a plane:

'In the unlikely event of a sudden loss of cabin pressure, oxygen masks will drop down from the panel above your head...Secure your own mask before helping others.'

Self-care means taking care of yourself first, so you can be of service to others. A quick google search of the term 'self-care practices' returns millions of articles and the variety of results include self-care practitioners, courses, podcasts, articles, books, YouTube channels, documentaries, websites, coaches and influencers. In fact, 4 840 000 000 results are retuned in 0.43 seconds. As much as self-care has become a trend, the number one self-care practice you can have in your life is sobriety.

What is self-care?

In the book *Creating a place for self-care and wellbeing in higher education*, edited by Narelle Lemon, self-care is defined as 'a multidimensional, multifaceted process of purposeful engagement in strategies that promote healthy functioning and enhance well-being'. It is a conscious act a person can take to promote their own physical, mental and emotional health. When it comes to equipping yourself to live out your best life, self-care is vital as it helps build resilience towards the stressors in life that you can't control. You know, your boss being a jerk, that guy cutting you off in traffic, spilling your coffee on your crisp white shirt or your footy team losing the Grand Final. For some, self-care can be misinterpreted as a luxury rather than a priority. This can lead to denying yourself of care as it conjures up feelings of guilt. However, self-care doesn't need to be a six-week holiday at The White Lotus. It can simply be a daily five-minute practice to help you handle life's inevitable challenges and manage your load effectively without overwhelm. For many, drinking started as the self-care menu choice, yet it led to self-destruction.

> **... self-care is vital as it helps build resilience towards the stressors in life that you can't control.**

Do you feel like you're always running out the door and forgetting your keys? I feel you. If you're in my situation — you work full time; you have a young family; you're trying to 'gentle parent', which makes you want to snap; you're doing the juggle, the pivot and the balance all at once — time for self-care doesn't make it on the list easily. In seasons of high pressure and high stress, self-care can be sitting in the car for five minutes and breathing slowly, giving yourself a moment to recalibrate or listening to a beautiful song. It can be scribbling three things you love in your journal. Or giving yourself a hug. I am a big self-hugger. It works for me. Singing loudly when no-one can hear or dancing when no-one is watching. It's stealing a moment away from the distractions, for just you. The list is endless when it comes to options on how to give yourself a little bit of love. Self-care is about putting your whole focus on yourself just for a moment — and sobriety is the ultimate self-care practice. The compounded benefits of the time you give back to yourself by being sober, the peace it offers you, the calm and the clarity are all elements of self-care expressed through the one simple act of not drinking.

> *It's not just the 'not drinking' that is the self-care; it is what the 'not drinking' enables you to do. I don't need to do the big time-out self-care as much now I'm sober because I'm doing the daily self-care consistently and on the regular ... I'm so much more consistent at my workouts and yoga. I'm consistent with my food and making good, healthy choices that nourish me. I'm consistent with my sleep and it's not disrupted by the effects of alcohol. I can listen to my body more easily and know when it needs a break.*
> **Libby McMichael, yoga teacher**

Choosing not to put a toxic substance in your body, choosing not to drink to reward yourself, choosing not to lose yourself because you can't deal, choosing not to drink because life is tricky, or a day has been long or your kids are driving you mad or you hate your job or your hair or your clothes or your boss ... Choosing not to drink alcohol is self-care because you are choosing *you*. Some of the benefits of sobriety are immediate and some are invisible, and over time the compounded benefits of not drinking are a complete self-care practice.

Sobriety is self-worth

My drinking abilities were something I was praised for. I could keep up with the boys and kick it with girls. I could make friends in any given social scenario with a drink in my hand. As I was always up for a good time, and a night out, I became a permanent place on any invitation list. This kept my calendar full, my week busy and my feelings supressed. Being a social butterfly with booze at every turn was the key to my popularity. However, sobriety was the key to my self-worth. Alcohol might promise you status, recognition, acceptance and validation, but sobriety is the key to finding your true self-worth. There are many different terms we use to explain how we feel about ourselves: there's self-esteem, self-compassion, self-acceptance, self-respect, self-confidence and self-love. But the most vital concept of self is self-worth.

About self-worth

Self-worth is having a positive view about yourself and a feeling that you are a good person who deserves good things. It is at the core of our very selves — our thoughts, feelings and behaviours are intrinsically linked to how we view our worthiness and value as humans. There are a lot of misconceptions about what creates our self-worth, so here I have listed the items on the life list that are sometimes twisted into our definition of our self-worth but do not define it completely:

- *Accomplishments*: Kicking goals is great and it feels good to tick things off a list, but it doesn't have a direct relationship with your worth.

- *Age*: You aren't too young or too old. Your age is simply a number.

- *Bank balance*: Whether it's zero or has a lot of zeros, your wealth is not your worth.

- *Popularity*: Your value as a human isn't reflected in how large or intimate your friendship circle is. The quality of your relationships is what's important.

- *Opinions*: Whether it be an informed opinion, educated guess or speculation, what you think, say or do in response to the world circling around you doesn't equate to your worth.

- *Relationship status*: Single, dating, married, divorced or otherwise — again, it's quality that is the key.

- *Taste*: It doesn't matter if you like fancy things or are a fashion fail, your worth is the same regardless of the way you wear your fedora.

- *Tricks*: Your ability to do the splits is a great party trick, but it doesn't reflect your value.

- *Virality*: Follows, likes, retweets or how viral your latest video went has no impact on your innate value.

- *Work*: It doesn't matter what you do. Making sure you do it well and it fulfills you is more important.

If you believe you are worthy and valuable, you are worthy and valuable. If you don't have this belief about yourself, then this is something we can work on together. Increasing self-worth can be tricky. Here is a simple guide to get you started on your self-worth position.

1. Write down an affirmation and stick it anywhere you look: the fridge, your computer, the mirror. Repeat it regularly. For example, *I am enough, worthy of friendship and love, just as I am*.

2. Learn to accept a compliment. Saying thank you and acknowledging it will reinforce something positive in your mind, creating a positive self-talk feedback loop.

3. Look at the above list of what does not determine self-worth and remind yourself that these things do not place value or worth on you as a person. These things are great to have, to identify with and to explore, but they do not equate to your own self-worth. Hopefully you will have a feeling of relief when you can let go of the outer things that can sometimes mess with our self-worth. Your worth comes from within.

4. Work on identifying, challenging and externalising the inner critic, the voice that comes in and disrupts your peace: the not good enough, do better, comparison narrative that can become our internal dialogue. Become acutely aware that the inner voice is spruiking false-talk, and remind yourself, *you are worthy and valuable regardless of what you do or don't do.*

Sobriety will give you the clarity and self-care tools to start to understand fully your value, which is not attached to outside elements.

Your worth comes from within.

Sobriety is letting go

Let it go!

Let it go!

I know you just sang that in your head. Even if you don't have little ones, you know those words, that pitch, and you know you want to hit the high note. Letting go of things we think are working for us can be difficult. At this point, alcohol is a big enough deal for you to be letting go of it, but along with letting go of alcohol will come an opportunity to let go of some of the things that are associated with your drinking behaviour also. You don't need to change everything today. Just relax. But over the next few weeks some things will come up for you, and a reassessment of them might be in order. Let me explain what I mean, by showing you what came up for me.

Sober curiosity was so conflicting because I landed in a pattern of wanting to stop drinking — saying I wouldn't drink but then not having the strength to say no to the crowd and I would end up drinking again. I was so afraid to let go of my social status. I didn't want anyone to ask me what was wrong with me, so I kept drinking and going out even though internally I felt done for so long. It was a long year, and it took a while, but eventually I accepted that yes, my social life might blow up in my face and people might judge me, but I couldn't keep doing this anymore. I let go of what other people would think of me, and I realised you can't control anyone anyway. So, the self-torture and the blame-shame cycle I was trapped in were my own doing. People will do, say and think how they will, and you can't change that. You can only change you. So, I accepted that my social life might end up being a distant memory and I was okay with that. And do you know what happened? My life got so much better. Yes, I stopped going out to bars and drinking with people, but I found a whole new way to do life that was fulfilling and fruitful. What I was willing to let go of has come back around in my life in the most positive and satisfying way. I am present, in concrete relationships that I cherish and that nourish me. I am engaged, I remember and I feel whole. I had to let go of the opinions of others and embrace my own narrative. I decided to tell my story and become the author of my life.

> *I let go of trying to moderate. I realised that my sweet spot did not exist within the paradigm of moderation and that I needed to start living without alcohol for an indefinite period. Once I'd made this shift, I felt a huge sense of relief. A weight had lifted, and I felt positive, energised and excited about the future.*
> **Kathryn Elliott — alcohol coach and breast cancer survivor**

Let's kick it back to the old school to demonstrate this point. And by old school, I mean ancient tribes, way before the '90s, which feels a bit old school these days. There is a parable, a story, about a monkey known as 'The Monkey's Fist'. Ancient-day native tribes would set up monkey traps (I know, poor monkeys). They would use a hollowed-out coconut shell tethered to a tree. The coconut shell was filled with rice and beans and had a hole in it. The idea was, that a monkey would place its open hand in the shell to get the rice and beans, but the hole would not be big enough for a closed fist to get out of the shell. The monkey became trapped. But it wasn't the coconut that was trapping the monkey, it was what was in the monkey's fist that the monkey was unwilling to let go of. Ouch!

So, what are your rice and beans?

What are you hanging onto? Is it your image? Your status? Your friendships? Opinions? It might be the perception of what alcohol does for you, how it makes you feel or the abilities it gives you. Or perhaps it's what your friendships might look like without alcohol that keeps you at the bar. The unknown can be intimidating, but this is your opportunity to do some self-reflection and have a think about what you are hanging onto that is keeping you entwined with alcohol. In sobriety you will find the strength to let it go and the reward will come. When the monkey let go of the rice and beans, the reward was freedom, baby.

> *I love my life. I am so lucky. I survived it. I didn't ruin it. I have seen family members who have ruined it, and they are so miserable and resentful and angry. I can let go of the shit and hold onto the joy and not have to drink to numb the pain anymore and I can enjoy every moment. I am so grateful for the opportunity to grow.*
> **David Campbell — TV host, performer, dad**

Sobriety is dealing

Up until now it's fair to say that you might have been coping, or barely coping. You have been doing your best to navigate life. You might have done it well or terribly — it's not for me to guess or for you to feel bad about. You've done the best you can with the resources available to you, alcohol being the most frequently used coping mechanism.

Coping is a struggle, and struggling is the opposite of thriving. Coping is not the state of play for optimum life kick-assery. Coping means surviving. It can conjure up pictures of someone struggling to get enough air, reacting poorly, floundering about barely being able to keep their head above water and gritting their teeth until their molars split. Coping keeps you reactionary. Not responsive.

Dealing with your situation means effective progression and is the substance of optimal life kick-assery. By dealing with situations, you become aware of your emotions and your environment and can effectively process your circumstance. Dealing with a situation or an emotion means responding to it well. It is a doing word and involves acting, moving forward. It's progressive, not static. It's the ability to see a thing for what it truly is, take the necessary action and move into a new situation. This keeps you responsive.

When life gave you lemons, you are probably accustomed to getting out the tequila. But as this book is about living without alcohol, your new strategy about life giving you lemons can be to make lemon meringue pie.

A quick reminder:

- A *reaction* is an emotional, knee-jerk, fly-off-the-handle, often irrational, emotionally charged approach.

- A *response* is a calculated, logical, practical, controlled and balanced approach. Using the law of cause and effect, a universal belief states that each action produces a reaction, regardless of circumstance. A response will garner a better effect than a reaction.

When I started my sobriety, it wasn't a light or easy decision. It was planned, calculated — it was something I'd thought about for months. I obsessed over what it might look like for me: how bored I might be, which friends would ridicule me. At the time, the idea of sobriety was overwhelming and impossible, and I struggled to see how it was going to work. What I discovered early on was that I engaged in a response mechanism rather than a reaction mechanism to anything life threw at me. And in 2015 the curve balls came hard and fast. Even when I hit a personal crisis, I had the ability to navigate it well.

Matt's story

Dr Matt Agnew, science communicator and author, took some time away from alcohol after he found himself in a dangerous cycle and depressed state.

'At the start of 2020, I had a very public break-up. Break-ups alone obviously are hard enough but throw on top of that the additional layer of public commentary and criticism and it became a really hard situation to navigate. It weighed on me very heavily. Some of the nastiness and vitriol slung my way really stung and it was a bit of a case of being kicked repeatedly while I was down.

Beyond that I had several other bumps in the road, which led to a slow but perceptible decline in my mental health that correlated strongly with an increase in alcohol consumption. Obviously, that led to a dangerous feedback loop: alcohol helped in the short term, but — being a depressant — it then led to an even more depressed mood the next day, which led to more alcohol … and so the cycle continued. It all sort of popped in February 2020 when I overindulged at two weddings and fell into a tremendously dark and dangerous state of mind.'

All the feels

It is evidenced by so many stories and overwhelmingly enthusiastic reviews that sobriety will have a positive impact on your physical wellbeing, and the benefits aren't limited to just your physical self. There are equally as important benefits to your emotional health, including emotional stability and emotional regulation, which can impact everything: from your relationships, to motivation and to your general mood. So, get ready for those feelings.

In general, you are more emotionally stable, connected and balanced without swigging booze. You already knew that though, and just to clarify, sobriety doesn't autocorrect a bad day, a crappy mood or a less-than-awesome event in your life. The rollercoaster of life still rolls on. The curveballs keep coming. The surprises, delights and disappointments will play out, but what sobriety offers you is the best chance of navigating these hurdles and overcoming them successfully without substance dependence. Sobriety gives you quality control over your physical, mental, emotional and brain health. The emotional benefits of sobriety can be evidenced in:

- increased confidence
- emotional stability
- better overall wellbeing
- improved relationships
- more motivation
- depression relief
- anxiety relief.

Sign me up!

Bex's story

Bex Weller, founder of Sexy Sobriety and the clipboard queen in her social group of friends, was always up for a good time and night out until she realised she wanted to stop drinking for a bit. Bex explains how she felt after having her last drink.

'For me, the wheels had been coming off for a while. I knew I needed some time off alcohol, but I was terrified to stop. The usual fears of how I will celebrate and how I will relax were very present. So I decided to bid farewell to alcohol for one last time. I drove an hour south to visit my parents at their house. I hadn't told anyone what I was considering. I started drinking, as we usually did, but this time, the whole night was tinged in sadness. I drank myself into a blackout and woke up in their spare room. That morning, I told my parents I was taking a break from drinking. I hadn't yet told my partner, and as I drove home, I just sobbed. I was so upset with myself for not stopping earlier. It felt like every emotion came flooding to the surface. As I arrived home, though, I began to feel relieved, and the first flurry of hope that things could be different.'

Personally, I went into sobriety quite clueless but with an open mind. Much like how I went into General Pants to find myself a new outfit when I was in high school, or how I went into my first *MTV* audition with my hair in half pigtails. In the very early days of sobriety three things became very clear to me and they were all quite unexpected. I had little idea of the process I was undertaking. This is not to say each person will have the exact same experiences in early sobriety as I did, but I would have appreciated a heads up, so here's yours:

1. Expect to feel super tired in the early evenings.

2. Expect your sugar cravings to go through the roof.

3. Expect to feel like crying, heaps.

The best thing to do if these sobriety symptoms present themselves is to honour them. Go to bed early, have an ice cream and sit with your feelings. Perhaps not in that exact order. Allowing yourself to experience what you are experiencing will be a new skill you learn in early sobriety. Honouring what you need, be it rest or a big cry, is okay. You are allowed to give yourself what you need. You are probably accustomed to ignoring how you feel and denying yourself of what you truly need, using alcohol as a numbing agent. I understand this feeling business might be new, and uncomfortable, but sit in it. It's good for you. Feelings are like a game of neighbourly knock and run. You hear them; you open the door with a slight panic and realise it's nothing. It's gone. And hopefully there isn't a bag of poo lit on fire on your doorstep. Although to be fair, processing feelings can resemble this *Billy Madison* movie moment at times.

Let's switch gears now.

Activity: a moment of gratitude

Write a letter to yourself expressing how grateful you are for arriving at this crossroads and acting. Tell yourself that it's okay: the past is forgiven, you are managing the present, micro-adjusting and the future looks heavenly. This is a self-care exercise and gratitude double whammy! Love and gratitude are nurturing for your soul. Here are some thought starters:

+ I am grateful for my breath.
+ I am grateful for today.
+ I am grateful for my future health.
+ I am grateful for the sun.
+ I am grateful for this book.
+ I am grateful for my willingness to learn new habits.
+ I am grateful for my choices.
+ I am grateful for the changes I am consciously making.

For so many years you know I really did think that one day I would wake up and just stop drinking. But that didn't happen. Not even after those mornings when I woke up so hungover and embarrassed about the night before that I swore I wouldn't drink again. Not even after I felt shame and guilt for my inability to cope with my life. Not even after I tried so hard. Not even after a Dry July. The divorce. The new job. Not even when I turned 30, or 34. Not even when I manifested another dream job. Not even when I met my favourite bands (Foo Fighters, Good Charlotte, Fall Out Boy) or my favourite actress (Sandra Bullock) or famous comedians (Chris Rock, pre-slap, Amy Schumer, Amy Poeler) or when I met my favourite pop stars (Lady Gaga, Katy Perry, Robbie Williams, 1D), or when I interviewed Sir Richard Branson, or partied with the Black-Eyed Peas. Or when I was serenaded by The Script, chilled with The Red Hot Chili Peppers or celebrated Occy's 40th, The Veronicas' 21st, visited Japan with Jason Mraz, or went on safari in South Africa. I jumped out of planes, heli-boarded, bungee-jumped, drove monster trucks, rode rollercoasters, swam with sharks, surfed in Spain, got lit in Las Vegas and danced in Dubai. There were so many 'pinch myself moments' in my career, and I thought that one of them would be big enough for me to overcome my alcohol dependence. It didn't make a difference how incredible the outer experience of my life was. How wonderful the stories, the moments or the memories were. How exclusive or exciting the rooms I was in were, or how popular and pretty the people I met were. My struggle with alcohol use was an inside issue. I only overcame it when I realised what I was doing wasn't sustainable for optimum life kick-assery, and so I made a change. But first, I made a plan. I am a planner.

My struggle with alcohol use was an inside issue.

I woke up one day, after months of planning and years of alcohol abuse, and made an incredibly confronting and challenging conscious decision to not drink alcohol regardless of what happened. I have made that same choice every day since. The choice is easier now because I understand myself better than ever, and I have the tools I need to deal with life: its ups and downs, curveballs and unfairness. When I first stopped drinking, my plan was to go without booze for a month and see how it looked, and a few months later, it was looking great, so I kept going. I was doing what was working for me, and sobriety was working so well. Some days were harder than others, but I felt so good. I looked so good, but was I ever going to drink again? This was a question I was asked a lot in the first few months of sobriety. And at the time I wasn't totally sure … until I *was* totally sure I wouldn't. The realisation that I was done with drinking came in the form of a complex intertwining of brutality and beauty 10 months into my sobriety. It was a moment I will never forget.

A few months into my not drinking stint, I had a conversation with a work colleague who asked me if there was something that 'would make me drink again'. She was curious about my sober curiosity. I hadn't said to myself, or anyone else for that matter, I was never drinking again but it had certainly been long enough to garner the question. My reply was something along the line of, 'Babe, the absolute worst thing in the world that could possibly happen to me at this point in life, would be if I lost my job. I love this job so much and I've worked seven years to get here, so maybe if I lost my job, I might drink again. Maybe.'

I guess I'm not going to drink again

In 2015, I started hosting the *Sydney Breakfast Show* on 2day FM. I also stopped drinking that same year. That big-deal radio job that Mark had put on my radar seven years earlier had manifested. The breakfast show was broadcast on the radio station I listened to growing up. I was sitting in the very chair my radio idol Wendy Harmer had sat in when I was a kid. I was talking into that microphone. I was doing that job. The dream.

It was a big, stressful and at times overwhelming job *and I was doing it sober*. But boy was it fun — so much fun! I had let go of drinking and maintained my position in media. I was doing the radio gig I had always wanted, and I was doing it fully sober, fully present and at full speed ahead. It was exhilarating and exhausting.

I cruised through my birthday in March. I signed up for Dry July to keep myself accountable. I sailed into September. All sober. Doing a live show each weekday morning, waking up in my hometown of Sydney, playing pop music and interviewing my favourite stars. Now I was the girl from the radio. My job was my identity: the ruler of my schedule and my life. I loved it and alcohol wasn't anywhere in the picture. In the past, to cope with the load of a loaded career, I would drink. Somehow drinking offered me control, until I couldn't control it any more, so the switch to sobriety gave me control again. Sobriety was my superpower. And it felt so good. I looked so great. I had started working out instead of frequenting after-work drinks. My head was clear. I felt truly joyful. Finally my life was on point and not just on paper. I was on billboards and my career was on fire, in a good way. Until the 6th of October 2015.

Let's back track slightly.

I had been sent on assignment to Austin, Texas by Red Bull Australia to be the Aussie correspondent at a music festival. Tough gig, huh? After finishing my field-reporting duties and catching the Foo Fighters show, I flew home to Sydney to get back to my breakfast radio gig. I had taken an additional day of leave to ensure I was recovered enough from the long-haul flight home. The plane landed just after 6 am in Sydney, and my plan was to head home, stay awake for the day and get back on the local time as I had a show the following morning. Naturally, I switched on my phone to catch up on all the news as I waited to get off the plane. A text popped up from co-host Dan. It simply read 'LOL' with a link to a news article. I clicked on the link. The article that popped up on my screen was speculating former TV host Rove McManus was rumoured to take over the reins of the 2dayFM breakfast show in 2016. *LOL indeed*, I thought. I put it down to fake news and got off the plane. The breakfast show was *my* job and I loved it. I felt comfort in knowing I was only 10 months into a two-year radio deal. I grabbed my luggage and got in a cab.

At 10 am, just as I had come back from a morning swim to keep myself awake, I received a phone call. It was two of the senior executives from the radio network. I answered the phone and joked, 'So, tell me the bad news bosses.' There was a brief, awkward silence. I assumed they were calling to tell me what a great job I did for Red Bull. Sadly, I was informed by the company execs that a new breakfast show had been signed for 2016. What the?!

I was thanked for my efforts during the year as it was made very clear that the Dan & Maz magic was done. The news article was spot on. My contract, as it would turn out, was not. I found out exactly who the incoming breakfast team was, like everyone else, a few days later via a shared story on my Facebook Newsfeed.

And I guess that was that.

I didn't know what to do. I had to go to work the next day and do a radio show as if everything was peachy in my world. We all put on a brave face and a great show and continued to do so until the final day when, without too much fuss, we quietly announced it was our last show. I cried. Of course, I cried. I was devastated. All the hard work, the late nights, the stress, the wins and talkability. It all added up to nothing in that moment. And this was the moment I said would drive me to drink. Despite my sadness, my disappointment, the public humiliation, being labelled a failure and a sacked radio star …

I didn't drink.

Looking back, I felt like I had navigated an intense and disappointing season with grace. Yes, I was upset. Like proper, crawl up into a ball and ugly cry devastated. Now, you might be thinking, 'Geez Maz, why so dramatic? It was just a job babe!' But wait, I had spent seven years working towards getting and keeping that job. The job was me! My identity was the job. My livelihood was the job. I was so interconnected to the job I didn't know who I was without it. So, when I lost my job, I felt like I lost myself too.

But I didn't drink.

In fact, I didn't even think about having a drink.

I really didn't want our last show to end. I didn't want to walk out of that building with no assurance of self or future stability. I didn't want the dream to be over, but clearly it was. I had no plan in place if this job didn't last a decade. I thought I had found my path. It turns out, the path is crazy complicated. I made an appointment to see my therapist, which helped. You see, because I wasn't reaching for the familiar muti-tool of coping — that being booze, baby — which would lead me to wash away any feelings I didn't feel comfortable with, I was able to deal with and process my feelings. Even though this was a big kick in the ovaries, I was able to deal with it effectively. Talking to a professional helped me sit strapped into the emotional roller-coaster you go on when you suffer a loss, and I had chalked up a few significant ones over the years by then. It was in this moment I realised I wasn't going to drink again. I was so done. As was my career!

Drinking will temporarily dissolve the discomfort you're feeling but it will not change your circumstances.

Let's say you lose your job like I did. Or a relationship ends; your business fails; something unplanned, unexpected and not super cool happens. Your reaction in the past has been to drink to cope with the situation. When things are unfair or unexpected it's usually the first resort. It certainly was for me for a very long time. The general vibe is to go out and get blind, or go to a friend's house with a bottle of wine. Have you ever noticed though, that no matter how much you drink, you're not getting the job back? Drinking doesn't change the situation you are in. It doesn't fix it, reverse it or make it go away. A drink, or a few, will temporarily give you an ability to block out reality and skew your perspective. It's a distraction, not a solution. You drink, you cry, you carry on, you get angry. But by morning, when you wake up, you find yourself still fired from your job, or heartbroken or sad. And it still sucks. Drinking will temporarily dissolve the discomfort you're feeling but it will not change your circumstances.

When I lost my job, as upset as I was, I decided to *respond* with grace and style. I sent the incoming breakfast team a welcome gift in the new year, and I threw myself into some new things I had on the backburner. Up until then, my radio job had truly taken over my life but being unemployed gave me some extra hours in the day to do some stuff I'd always wanted to do. As scary as it was to be jobless and out of an industry I had hated to love for so long, I looked for the blessing. I found the silver lining. I started to rediscover myself.

And I didn't drink.

Once I hung up the headphones, I was given the gift of time and space to sit with myself and work out who I was away from the airwaves. I could think about what I wanted and how I could create a new path for myself. Much the same as the first step in this process was giving up alcohol, the next step for me was dealing with a big life thing that turned out to be a blessing.

Want to see the law of cause and effect at its best?

This is the beautiful full circle of this story. Five years later, in 2020, the very same radio network that had dumped me from the airwaves offered me a new breakfast radio show with a bigger audience reach: a Super Show. I said yes and Amen. And because I had that few years away from media to figure out my purpose, I now come to radio content curation from a place of grounded authenticity and inner peace. I am, I believe, the best I have ever sounded on-air because I know who I am, what I stand for and why I am here. Sure, I have bad days. We all have bad days, but I have them sober and I navigate them with grace and style, with a dash of self-compassion. My life didn't self-correct when I got sober, but I found the strength and self-care to steer the ship and remain steady.

My last drink was on a beautiful summer day. My husband wasn't home and one of my kids wanted to be dropped off at a friend's

place but I couldn't take them because I was drinking… We have a pool and I remember telling the kids they couldn't go in the pool because I couldn't focus. When your kids are in the pool, you need to be able to look out for them, and I couldn't. So that was the reason why I stopped. I needed to be able to get in the car, look out for my kids and be a good mum, instead of sitting on the steps of my wine cellar drinking Penfolds Bin 29.
Irene Falcone — founder, Sans Drinks

Summing up …

+ Sobriety is a superpower: the longer you spend in sobriety, the easier it will become, and the knock-on compound benefits of sobriety really are endless.

+ Sobriety delivers on the promises that alcohol makes.

+ Sobriety is the ultimate self-care tool.

+ Sobriety will give you a renewed sense of self-worth.

+ To gain your complete self in sobriety you may need to let go of some of the expectations you've had and perceptions you've attached to alcohol and its role in your life. This may include letting go of relationships that are not serving you.

+ Sobriety gives you the space to feel your feelings and engage with your emotions, leading to better management of self-regulation.

+ Taking a moment, when you can, to be grateful is a good circuit breaker and can be grounding if your inner voice is getting too loud.

+ Be aware that you might love your sober life so much you won't want to give it up for anything, and that's a great thing.

Now you have some insight into what sobriety can look like, it's time to craft a Sober Toolkit and prepare you for your sobriety journey.

6 Your Sober Toolkit

Let's get you your very own, personalised Sober Toolkit. This chapter is full of practical tools and activities. It is important to have a clear intention for your sobriety and to equip yourself with tools that will guide your experience in sobriety. Safeguarding your sobriety is the goal here and this will set you up for success. Sobriety is not a fleeting five-minute pow-wow; it isn't a buy-one-get-one-for-free scheme; it's not on sale, but it's a good deal. Sobriety is your best chance at being your best self and all you need to do is simply not drink alcohol. The best way to access the tools you need to help you along the way is to collect them and keep them together in your own Sober Toolkit.

Before we personlise your Sober Toolkit there is one thing we need to drill down on. As I mentioned previously, writing is such an important part of this journey, and as you will see in Jay's story it can become a great source of processing, unpacking and redefining your relationship with alcohol. There are a couple of important activities, yes, that involve a bit of writing on your part. This will aid in your quest to draw a line in the sand, and embrace the alcohol reframe you have been learning about.

Jay's story

Jay Mueller, a world-class podcast producer and game-changer creative, wrestled with the impact his sobriety might have on his creativity and in turn his career. He explains that when he realised his relationship with alcohol was impacting his health severely, his immediate concern was connected to his identity in the media industry.

'I was immediately convinced that without drinking I was not going to be interesting or creative, and that no-one was going to call me for work any more. So, you know what I did? I did a lot of journalling and a lot of writing. All of it was just for me to try to sort through what I was going through and trying to figure out how I was feeling without alcohol. Writing can help you go just a little bit deeper, even if it's just one layer deeper, to try to figure out what the foundation is of that one feeling that you're at in the moment and being able to sit with it and work through it. It takes time and patience and I found it very rewarding.'

Jay's story identifies how you can begin to redefine your relationship with alcohol by journalling or writing.

Activity: a sobering letter

In part I you were able to define your relationship with alcohol through several important written activities. Now it's time to redefine your relationship with alcohol. What are you hoping this journey in sobriety will bring for you? A powerful way to do this is to write a goodbye letter to alcohol. Giving up alcohol can feel like a break-up. It's been a real relationship and it no longer serves you. Saying goodbye is a great way to mentally prepare for sobriety.

Writing a goodbye letter to alcohol

Remind yourself why your relationship with alcohol became complicated, unbalanced, too familiar or dangerous. Lay it all out. This is a big and important step in your journey. By being honest with alcohol, by accepting the part it has played in your life up until now, you are able to draw a line in the sand and choose differently. Farewelling this relationship may be a grieving process. It was for me. Love and grief are one and the same. You loved alcohol, or at least it served you at some point. It felt safe for you; it was your companion and your keeper of secrets until its destruction became overbearing. As with a toxic relationship, despite the pain, it may leave a gap when you say goodbye. Simply becoming aware of the impact saying goodbye will have, like any end to a relationship, will help you journey through the emotions that arise. Like a break-up, when you have spent all your time with someone, you miss them when they are not around — and you've been spending some significant time drinking, so you may miss it. Acknowledging alcohol's role in your world and explaining why you are moving on without it will be a fundamental part of the healing process.

Here are some thought starters:

+ What do you and alcohol do together?

+ How does alcohol make you feel?

+ What does alcohol offer to you?

+ What knock-on effect does your relationship with alcohol have?

+ What are the reasons you spend time with alcohol?

(continued)

- How much time do you spend with alcohol?

- Is this relationship working for you?

- What would your life look like without alcohol in it?

- How do you feel without alcohol?

- What are you scared of losing without alcohol in your life?

I'll go first.

Dear Alcohol,

We're done. I just can't do this anymore. I don't even understand why I can't seem to get by without you. You have a hold on me. I hate it. I push you away, then I come running after you. I have no idea how I am going to get through a day without you. I have become dependent. You have been the rock. You have been there through the drama, the trauma, the highs and the lows and I know I depend on you. I need you. And I hate it.

We used to be fun and exciting, but somewhere along the road, you became my ugly secret. My sole companion, my keeper of secrets, my vice and my undoing. You promised me an escape, confidence, numbness. You were sweet and innocent but now I am trapped. I am stuck. You have a hold and I can't seem to let go. You are breaking me. You are not good for me. You make things worse. How did this happen? I feel shame. I feel lonely. I am terrified to move on without you, but I cannot do this any more. I used to think I deserved you, but now I understand, I deserve so much more.

I am better than this. I am better than you. I do not know how, but this must end. I need to see who I am without you. Whoever I discover on the other side of this dependence, she needs me. I must find her and help her heal. I need to save her from this.

I used to think you would fix my problems, but you created more. I don't like what I do when I am with you. I don't like how you make me feel. You make me sick. I feel sad. You have robbed me of my memories, of my dignity, of my peace, of my purpose. I feel lost, I feel abandoned and I know I am the only one who can change this story. So, I am saying goodbye.

If I continue down this path, there is no escape. There is only a terrible end for me. I am spinning, I am spiralling. You are breaking me down. You crept in and took up residence, but I am kicking you out. This is my moment. This is the crossroads. Here at this junction. We are done.

I must have my last drink and see who I am without you.

And I hope she is amazing.

xoxo

Maz

Sober synopsis

In this section I will articulate an important piece of the sobriety puzzle by identifying a reason why you want to live without alcohol. By nailing down one good reason, you give yourself a built-in accountability to help keep you on the path to sobriety. A reason is a reminder for you in trying times that can keep you from a slip-up.

A reason

World renowned motivational speaker and not my guru Tony Robbins talks about finding something you want to live for that's bigger than yourself — a mission — all the time when we're having casual chats over brunch… *As if!* I *wish* I could have brunch with Tony Robbins. The closest I have come to Tony Robbins is being in the stadium at his 'Unleash the Power Within' event in 2018, at which there were two highlights:

- I was lucky enough to be in an aisle seat on the arena floor, up close to the action. The interaction came at the nine-hour point of day 1 and I was *exhausted*. My hands hurt from clapping, my voice was hoarse from yelling. Tony walked past my seat, and I waved my hand — a little wave from my lap. He pointed at me and nodded — like *I see you gurl*. At least that's my memory of the moment. Tony's subliminal validation gave me a second wind, which worked out well, as the second highlight was participating in the famous fire walk.

- We had spent the entire day — I'm talking 9 am to 9 pm — building up the mental tolls to complete the fire walk. Yes, walking barefoot across hot coals. Oprah's done it so I figured I could too. The build-up was so long and so intense, the moment was so quick and the aftermath was electric. Laid out in front of my bare feet were thousands of burning hot coals and I had only one way to get across them. I took a few deep breaths in and out and took a few quick steps as I yelled 'cool moss, cool moss, cool moss'.

I did not feel the fire. I felt like I had flown.

So, back to finding a good reason. In the lead-up to making the final decision to try sobriety, you may have been reflecting on why you haven't been able to get a grip on your drinking before now. You've tried moderation and it went okay for a few days or weeks but then you slipped back into the regular habit of drinking again.

Or maybe you have had a whole month off booze before but then after that, it's back to square one. Why is that? Are you trying to stop drinking for a little while to prove you don't have a problem? I tried that too.

With the information presented in this book, you now can articulate a solid purpose for your sobriety. Rather than overwhelm yourself by writing out lists of reasons and hundreds of apologies, let's just articulate one carefully thought-out reason why you are doing this. *Now is your opportunity to define what sobriety looks like for you.* Why do you want to make a shift that will be long lasting? Is it for your health? Your family? Your relationship? Your mental health? Whatever the reason, let's define it so you can use this to pull you towards sobriety, which, as Tony says, will be far more sustainable than pushing yourself.

As I shared earlier in this book, I had been looking for a reason to take some time away from drinking for months. I could feel my grip on my drinking habits slowly start to slip and I was looking for *any* excuse I could find to not be around people drinking, yet I failed every time to garner the strength to not go out and drink or to go out and not drink. I felt trapped in my own secret world of shame, and I didn't know where to seek out answers. I didn't think I needed AA because I had stopped drinking for an entire month in the past. Even though it felt like holding my breath for a month, I got through it only to end up counting down the minutes before allowing myself back in the same cycle of drinking. This time was different; there was a switch. I wanted to find my sober self and I was willing to let go of what I thought I knew to discover her. I arrived at a place where what I knew had stopped working for me. The nudge I needed happened to break my heart into a few thousand, tiny pieces, but I am grateful to this day for the grief which led me to my sober days.

David's story

David Campbell and I have circled around each other in the entrainment industry for two decades. We first met when he hosted VH1, which I used to refer to as 'the old person's *MTV*' as I was hosting *MTV* out of the same TV studios. David shared with me the reason bigger than him that led to him never having another drink.

'It's such a showbiz story. Dan Aykroyd had been in town promoting the new *Ghostbusters* and had handed out his Skull vodka. I was at home with my wife Lisa, and it was a Friday night. I thought, *we should open that bottle of vodka that Dan Aykroyd gave us, right?* And it was low key. We finished the bottle, and we had a few, but I don't remember being *drunk* drunk.

The next day we got up and I was so ill. We had to go to the airport. It was bad. We upgraded on points because I almost didn't get on the plane. I thought, *What is going on?* Then I heard Leo, my son, say, 'Oh, Dad's not well.' And that was the moment. I'd almost ruined our holiday. I'd almost not got my family to the plane. It was the knowledge of my son recognising that something had happened and Dad's not well. That is something I grew up around and I did not want to perpetuate that myth. I was done and that was my last drink.'

For me, the initial disbelief and shock of one of my closest friend's death sent me straight to the bottom of a bottle. It took me weeks of mourning Mark's death before I finally checked in to see a therapist to deal with my grief. It was there, on a little blue couch surrounded by lots of tissues, that my therapist and I came up with a way to move through the grief rather than circle around it. This was my *one good reason*, and it was bigger than me. Honouring Mark's life and making him proud was a bigger-than-me reason to go and try sobriety, and to try to navigate the grief I was journeying through without alcohol. I didn't want to dance around it anymore. I didn't want to white knuckle it again. I was tired of failing. Something had to change. And so, I made the change. Exploring sobriety felt rebellious, and I liked it. I felt like I was in control again, like I had a power move.

A superpower!

You must find another purpose, a focus, something that is bigger than yourself. I ended up joining a triathlon club. This was the game changer. I can honestly say fitness saved my life. I got into a half ironman. It took two and a half years. I was training, racing. I had a new focus, something to do. More importantly, I created a whole new version of myself.
Action Alexa — motivation/fitness expert

You have quite possibly been circumnavigating sober curiosity for some time. It keeps coming up for you. You keep reading about it, hearing about it, it's being signposted for you. The universe speaks to us in whispers: *Are you listening?* You can simply draw a line in the sand, rather than find the bottom of a brown paper bag. (If you shop at a wholefoods store and buy your grains in bulk you will use a lot of brown paper bags, so no offence if this is you.) Walking across a line in the sand is much easier than climbing out of the bottom of the ball pit. And on that note, why can't adults jump in the ball pit at kids' play centres. They are the best. We need to rethink that rule in society. A line in the sand. A simple empowered choice. A crossroads. A sliding doors moment.

I asked my husband about what he thought might have happened if he or I didn't stop drinking when we did, and he said he highly doubts our marriage would have lasted. I am so grateful for our collective sobriety; it's secured our relationship and it's become the best choice we made.
Libby McMichael — yoga teacher

WHAT YOU THINK IS YOUR REALITY

Whether it's true or a complete lie, it's still your truth because it's what you believe. Our perception is our reality. Anchor down and find your bigger purpose. Is it your kids? Your health? To save your relationship? To end your relationship? To do things differently from how your parents did? To challenge yourself? To see life through a brand-new lens? To save enough money to go overseas? To save enough money to help a family in need?

Be brave and commit to *one reason* big enough to give this sobriety thing a red-hot crack.

> *The very reason that I was drinking myself into oblivion became the new purpose in my life. My drinking unlocked the moment I knew I needed to stop and what I have built from there is so great, and so impactful. Sobriety gave me everything I ever wanted.*
> **Irene Falcone — founder, Sans Drinks**

A support system

After I googled 'Am I an alcoholic?' I came to the abrupt conclusion that I wasn't but that alcohol wasn't working for me. I sat with my reality, in a quiet room, and wrestled with my feelings. After crying a lot, I called my mum. Mum and I have always been close. She is one of the kindest and wisest people I have ever known. She is gracious, compassionate, honest and deeply loving. She also uses emojis to communicate entire conversations over text and doesn't like driving at night these days. She's my mum. And I was so afraid to tell her my truth. I had hidden it well; no-one knew the inner workings of suffering I was grappling with behind the shiny radio job and endless amounts of praise I received. I wanted to tell my mum because I knew I needed her support. But I was worried about how she would react. I explained to Mum on the phone — after some self-reflection, a few counselling sessions and a recycling bin full of empty wine bottles — that I was dependent on alcohol, and that I was planning on doing something about it. My heartbeat got a little louder in the moment after I said out loud, 'I have a problem with alcohol' in anticipation of her reaction. She responded with compassion. Despite my mum's complete shock at my admission, at no point did I feel judged. I felt loved.

The next person I called was my boyfriend (now husband). Again, I explained my conclusion and the plan of planning my sobriety. I was met with acceptance, care, kindness and support about my sober exploration. I was listened to, I felt heard, space was held for me, I felt seen. I came undone, I felt safe. The reality hit me when I said it out loud, and the support I was offered cemented my decision. It was happening. I finally felt a sense of relief. I had identified the crossroads, drawn the line in the sand. And now I could get to work. There were two important people I told when I planned to stop drinking and they became my sober support system. And even in the first few weeks, I didn't really talk about it with anyone else. I just got on with it. I kept my head down, I ordered soda water and I went home early. But I was able to discuss how I was feeling, what I was going through and what was coming up for me with my mum and my boyfriend.

Your drinking buddies are not going to be your support system here, I'm sorry to say. You'll need to reach out beyond the bounds of your social drinking friends to find a support and accountability partner for this season of sobriety.

Yumi Stynes, media personality and supermum, opened up on the *Last Drinks* podcast about her experience of attending her first AA meeting and how revolutionary that decision was for her moving forward with her sobriety journey after a previous slip-up on day 4.

It took a huge amount of courage to admit I am a broken human who needs some help, and it feels like you're putting your reputation on the line, which I think is fair to everyone, whether or not they work in the public eye. But in just one meeting I suddenly felt like being accountable is going to really help me.
Yumi Stynes — sober since 2014

Like many things in life, sobriety is going to be an easier journey with support. You have the support of the sobriety tools in this book to lean on, but you may also need additional support. As much as sobriety is a superpower, you don't need to be a superhero about it and try to do it all alone. It takes a village. It's up to you how you engage support. My recommendation is to find what works for you. It might be a counsellor, a friend, a sober coach, an online support group or something else completely. Finding someone to help you keep accountable, someone to unpack the tough stuff with and celebrate the wins with is going to make this experience a more impactful one for you. My personal advice is to only tell who you need to at first and get them on board with your plan. *If you don't have friends and family nearby, or if you need more support, you can refer to the list of sober support services in the references section at the end of this book.*

Like many things in life, sobriety is going to be an easier journey with support.

A response

People will want to know why you are not drinking. People are so nosy. They will want answers, and only answers that they are happy with. Now, to be fair, it really isn't their business why you decided to stop drinking, but it is wise to have a way to respond to the quick-fire questions. Crafting a sober response will help you prepare for and navigate social events and family interactions in early sobriety. You know why you are not drinking. You are clear on your commitment. A sober response is the statement you can make to anyone who questions your sobriety. Please do not apologise for being sober. I did this a lot in early sobriety. If someone offered me a drink, I would reply with, 'Oh no, sorry, I'm not drinking right now.' This reply felt weak, like I wasn't sold on my own sobriety journey; that I was being an inconvenience. I soon realised that I wasn't in fact sorry for my choice not to drink alcohol, so I started to own it and my reply turned into, 'No, I'm good thanks.' I felt more secure in this response. I felt like it was a power move. I was more than okay with my decision not to drink alcohol for a period, and I felt empowered communicating it with a splash of oomph.

Most of us overshare and say way too much when asked about why we are not drinking. Here is what you say if someone asks you if you want a drink. You say, 'No thanks. I'm not drinking these days. I'll have a water.' That's it! If you get a follow-up question, which usually you won't, respond with, 'It was affecting my sleep so I'm taking a break.' And then stop talking.
Belle Robertson — sober coach and author, *Tired of Thinking About Drinking*

Some people are kind-hearted creatures, and others are flat-out jerks. Here are some interactions I had in early sobriety. Let these be an encouragement for you to drill down on your sober response:

- *Did something happen?* Nothing happened, I am just having a break from alcohol.

- *Did you have a drinking problem?* I just want to have a break from alcohol. It's not working for me.

- *When will you start drinking again?* I'm not sure. Watch this space. I feel amazing.

- *Why don't you just have one?* I challenged myself to do zero drinks for a period and I want to achieve that goal. So none is good, thanks.

- *But it's my [insert celebration here].* I'm here celebrating with you. Let's dance. I'm here to have a good time and I can do that without drinking.

- *C'mon, just have one.* I don't want to. My promise to myself is too important.

- *Oh, so you're too good for us now?* Our relationship is stronger than our drinking sessions. Why don't we go for a walk early one morning and catch up properly.

- *Does this mean I can't drink around you?* If I feel uncomfortable, then I'll go home. But you carry on. I'm not asking you to stop. I'm just asking you to support my decision.

- *You're so boring.* I haven't changed as a person; I'm just not drinking. What would be great as my friend, would be if you could support my decision.

- *What are you going to do every weekend?* My plan is to get up early and make the most of the day. I'm busy doing *new* things. I'm excited to see how that plays out.

- *Did you join a cult?* No, sobriety isn't a cult. Scientology might be?

- *What's wrong. Why aren't you drinking?* Oh wow, I love your shoes. Are they new? (People love talking about themselves. I love asking questions. Deflect the conversation to another topic.)

- *Are you pregnant?* Both men and women get asked this question. If a man isn't drinking it might be assumed his partner is pregnant. If a woman isn't drinking it might be assumed she is with child. This is a complex topic, especially for some men and women who have had a complex journey with fertility. I know what that is like. As this is a sensitive topic, my suggestion would be to say as little as possible if you are uncomfortable discussing it and change the topic or excuse yourself to get a glass of water.

Sober power moves

Have a think about the moments and situations that pop up and leave you wanting that drink. Think about those situations and how you can adopt some simple power moves to reframe those moments and keep you accountable to your sober decision.

Out to dinner:

- Order sparkling water for the table.
- Take the wine glasses off the table or turn them upside down.
- Return the drinks menu.

In a bar:

- Always keep a fresh glass of water in one hand.
- Remember your sober response.
- Go home early.
- Have a plan for early the next morning.
- Be the designated driver.
- Order food.

At a social event. As above plus:

- Stay on the dance floor.
- Take your own alcohol-free drinks.
- Offer to organise some games to play: old school croquet, reflex tennis, volleyball, frisbee, hopscotch (although the name of this last one may be triggering for some).

At home:

- Throw away all your alcohol.
- Keep plenty of herbal tea in the cupboard.
- Buy a soda stream.
- Keep healthy snacks on hand in the fridge and pantry.
- Have a friend to call as a support person if you feel like having a drink.
- Start a new hobby to keep your hands occupied.
- Buy a massage gun and treat yourself to home massages.

By yourself:

- Do some breath work.

- Go for a walk; change your environment.

- Go to bed early.

- Have a cup of herbal tea.

Having some strategies in place so you're prepared if you're tempted by alcohol is going to make this ride a bit easier. You'll know what to do if you unexpectedly find yourself at an event where alcohol is being served. It is wise to pre-think these situations, so you have a premeditated response. It is my advice to avoid any triggers as you navigate early sobriety. This may mean keeping your social calendar empty for a few weeks, although it is more than possible to stop drinking one day and attend a hen's party the next, as Bex Weller, founder of Sexy Sobriety, explains.

I told my love, 'This is going to be my day 1' and he was like, 'That's wonderful. Finally. But don't you have a hen's party to go to tomorrow?' I did. It amped up the anxiety, that's for sure, but the relief of knowing things were going to be different this time helped me get through it. When I arrived at the hen's party, I must admit, it was incredibly awkward. I'd always been the biggest drinker in our social group, but this time I'd actually driven to the party. I bolted over to the drinks to grab myself an OJ as soon as I arrived. A friend asked if I was driving, and I mumbled yes and that I was taking a break from drinking.

A goal

If you are a ticking-off-lists, goal-oriented person, then adding in a goal for this season of sobriety might be an additional strategy to help you through. I am talking about the goal-setting theory. Setting yourself a personal goal is a way to influence your behaviour and add some incentive into your sobriety plan. I understand that being sober is your focus, but personally I found early on, my thought loops became focused, almost obsessed on *not having a drink*. I thought a lot about 'not drinking'. It consumed my thoughts because it was what I was trying *not to do*. Sometimes distraction is a great tool. Having a clear goal in mind outside of your quest for sobriety can help you to stay motivated and will keep your mind away from thinking about drinking for the first few weeks of sobriety.

We've already done a few activities to help you identify what your relationship with alcohol is like. To continue this exploration, setting a goal is a great way to help keep you on your sober path during your time away from alcohol. Your goal needs to be specific, measurable, attainable, relevant and time-bound. The overarching goal in this scenario is to explore being sober for at least 30 days, but adding in a sober SMART goal is a great addition to help incentivise you to stick to your sobriety.

Here are some examples of sober SMART goals:

- Put any money I would spend on alcohol (specific; measurable) into a piggy bank (attainable) and then spend it on something I want (relevant) at the end of the month (time-bound).

- Use the time I would usually spend at the bar (specific; measurable) at the gym instead (relevant; attainable) and measure my body composition before and after 30 days (time-bound).

- Walk for 20 minutes (specific; measurable) each morning I am sober (relevant; attainable; time-bound).

- Write a page in my journal (specific; measurable) each night before I go to sleep (relevant; attainable) during my sobriety (time-bound).

I do not want this to become a pressure for you though. This might not be the right strategy for you. Don't overload yourself if this is too much, but if you like the idea of distracting yourself sober, then finding a goal for this time away from alcohol will give you an extra focus and something to work towards during this time. *Know thyself.* If this is your thing, go for it. And if it's not, then leave it out.

Activity: a sober synopsis

I want you to keep these next few activities together in one section of your journal where you can refer to them easily. This page is your sober synopsis, and it will safeguard you in early sobriety. This gives you a solid foundation to build your sobriety on.

Here is how it will read.

Sober response

Write down your sober response. Please be as succinct and as direct as possible.

Sober support system

List the handful of people you are going to share your sober plan with and ask for support. Write down how you will have the conversation and what you are asking of them. Give them your time frame and ask them to be your accountability partner.

Sober reason

Write in detail your one bigger-than-you reason for giving sobriety a go.

Sober goal

Make one goal for your time away from alcohol that isn't related to sobriety. Make it one thing to focus on and stick to the SMART goal-setting system.

Examples

Here are some examples of a sober response:

+ I'm taking a break from drinking.

- I'm not drinking tonight.

- I'm the designated driver.

- I'm good with water, thanks.

- I've got to get up early to go to the gym / get in my morning walk / do yoga / take an international conference call...

Here are some questions you can ask yourself to nail down one bigger-than-you reason why you want to explore sobriety:

- I wonder how epic my life can be?

- How fit can I get?

- How great can I feel?

- How can I help others?

- How can I be an inspiration?

Here are some goal ideas you can articulate into SMART goals to suit your needs:

- Start a daily yoga practice.

- Complete a fun run.

- Commit to a savings plan.

- Volunteer.

Remember, you can always go home early; you have permission to tap out and look after yourself. This sober journey is an exercise in giving you what you need, and you are allowed to prioritise your sobriety. So if it's all too much, go home — just don't have a drink. Get to bed early, then get up early and do something that makes you feel great.

This is your time to shine. This is your journey — your story — and only you can write it.

Your Sober Toolkit

Let's put together your personal Sober Toolkit. This is about finding the tools that work for you and utilising them. Try to cherry pick a few favourites, rather than overwhelm yourself by doing too many. Remember, sobriety is the key here. Adding in lots of new things all at once may feel like too much and lead you to undo the work you've started. My advice is, read about each sober tool: if it feels like 'you', pop it in your Sober Toolkit. While completing the Sober 30 (in part III of this book) you will be trying out a whole bunch of different activities, so you can grow your Sober Toolkit as you go. It's a progression.

Here are my sobriety tools.

Create a sleep schedule

Sleep is a recipe for mental, physical and emotional harmony. It can sharpen your memory; help your body heal; improve mood and muscle strength; and give your mental health a boost. Creating a sleep routine will help to optimise your sober self. You can simply start with a sleep wake-up time. Or go all in and create an entire sleep routine. *Go to sleep and wake up at the same time every day — yes, even on the weekend.* This will vary if you are a shift worker or a new parent, but the goal here is to do your best to get your head on the pillow and get out of bed at the same time each day. It will create a routine: we are creatures of habit, and we thrive on routine!

As we sleep in 90-minute cycles, you can try to time your sleep so you wake up at the end of a sleep cycle. To do this, figure out what time you need to be awake in the morning, and count back in 90-minute increments, giving yourself a minimum of seven hours' sleep. Then go to bed at that time and see if you wake up a little easier. For example, if you want to wake up at 6 am, 6 × 90-minute sleep cycles will have your head hitting the pillow at 9 pm. That's a total of up to nine hours' sleep.

Create a bedtime routine

I am a routine genie. I thrive when I am in a routine, which is probably why I was so into dance classes and trying to learn the 'Bye Bye Bye' N'Sync choreography when I was younger. Dance routines, daily routines, they both work for me. And yes, I also loved aerobics in the early 1990s just if you were wondering. There are a few key things you can fold into your end of and beginning of day that will create a bedtime routine to help optimise your sleep:

- taking magnesium an hour before bed, for muscle relaxation

- putting lavender essential oil in a diffuser

- turning off all screens two hours before bed, for mental relaxation

- listening to an end-of-day or body-scan meditation.

Stay hydrated

Keep a glass of water by your bedside. Water will kick-start your digestion on rising, eliminate that groggy first-thing-in-the-morning feeling, help flush out toxins and boost your immunity.

Normalise two glasses of water each morning — yes, before your coffee — and stay hydrated with water intake throughout the day. Why do we need to drink so much water? Well, we are made up of 70 per cent water, just like the planet we live on. You can go weeks without food, but only a few days without water. As you are used to drinking alcohol, water may feel a bit boring, but again, this is the time for new things, so find a way to enjoy getting your daily dose of hydration.

Have cold showers

This may sound wild to you, but I have a cold shower every morning. At first, I would spend at least two minutes psyching myself up to jump in. I would grab my opposite shoulders in a brace position and get under the freezing water while holding my breath and almost hyperventilating. And after 30 seconds I would jump out and wrap myself in a towel. But over time, after reading about the documented benefits of cold emersion therapy (including a 2021 *The Conversation* article by Lindsay Bottoms), I was able to spend less time psyching myself up for a cold shower in the morning and more time in the cold shower. And I love it now. I didn't love it at first, but it's a great way to wake yourself up in the morning. Or to give yourself a reset in the middle of a tough day.

Focus on food

As much as you can, get a good balance of proteins, vegetables and carbohydrates. Without going into too much detail here, a serving of protein should be the size of your hand. Your plate should be 60 per cent vegetables, and carbs should be minimal. Go for ancient grains over processed ones. Eat as much whole produce as possible and limit anything out of a box. Eat until you are 80 per cent full and then stop. This is all stuff your grandparents told you. I'm just putting it in for a quick reference. Find some healthy snacks and lean on them. And do your best to enjoy your food. So much of our modern diet culture is about deprivation. Look, if you're doing all the right things with your food choices for 80 per cent of the week, then you can have a cupcake one day. Just one — a fully sugar-filled, nasty one — and enjoy every bite. Being present with our food is a lost art and eating mindfully is a practice you can easily create each time you have a meal. Try not to eat or drink on the go. Be in the moment, mindful and grateful for the nourishment you are giving your body.

What is your food rule? I take mine from journalist and author Michael Pollen, who writes in his book *In Defense of Food*, 'Eat food. Not too much. Mostly plants.' This is not about adding to your load by giving you another chore to wrap your head around, but nutrition is key and when you have time — which you will when you're not drinking — it's a good idea to think about how you can nourish your body. Eating for fuel, cooking from scratch, and creating a practice around whole and healthful foods will help your body heal.

Exercise

Aim to move your body each day, especially if you have a rather sedentary day schedule. Working out at the gym is great if that works for you, but if not, there are some simple daily routines you can get your body into the swing of, like running, walking or swimming each day.

As a starting point, aim to walk 7000 steps a day.

Do some stretching on rising or before bed. A quick, five-minute sun salutation, or a longer routine if you have the time. There are millions of quick workouts online and there are thousands of apps for exercise. Again, this is about finding one exercise that you can stick to. If you hate the gym, *don't join a gym*. If you love running, *then run*. If you prefer to walk, *then walk*. Dynamic stretching is better than static stretching, so stretch for a few minutes in the morning by moving through the stretch. What is important is to do something every day, weekends included, so make it something you love and something you want to do. If you feel like a drink, do 20 star jumps. Try to touch your toes for two minutes or do a headstand. Being upside down can be a great reset.

Do some journalling

The power of the pen is one of my go-to tools and works wonderfully for the owner of an overactive mind. I journal in the middle of the night if my head is spinning, and it helps settle down the steady stream of thoughts swirling through my mind. You can journal about a moment, the past, your future, your feelings ... whatever.

You can make it a daily practice or use it as a go-to tool when you can't escape the thought loop. It's a circuit-breaker. Writing with a pen on paper is my recommendation. And take a note of the date and time: it might be helpful to reflect on your journey and give yourself some milestones for what you have been able to process, resolve and work through.

Meditate

Finding a meditation practice was tough for me. I have an endless feedback loop and constant stream of chatter in my mind. I am a chronic overthinker, and so meditation really isn't my strong suit. That said, I try. To be totally honest, I still struggle to find a daily practice of meditation; however, what I do notice when I have a good streak of meditative moments is that I feel calm. I feel centred and the thoughts do tone themselves down. A guided meditation is my go-to and 10 minutes is my maximum effort. Even a simple 10 minutes in the busy part of the day can reset the mental load. It's also a beautiful 'wind down at the end of a day' tool. A meditative body scan can settle me down ready for rest. As well, it's a great way to start the day by sitting with yourself and setting an intention for the day.

Find a mantra

Repeating a mantra can be useful as it employs the thinking mind instead of trying to ignore it or silence it. By repeating a mantra, you are using thoughts to transcend thoughts, which is extremely skilful. Simply repeating a mantra over and over in your head for a set period is a great tool. Find a few favourites, write them on notes and leave them where you will be able to read them: on your fridge, your mirror, your computer. In your office, at your desk, in your car, in your lunchbox, behind the toilet door.

I grow through what I go through.

My three mantras for sobriety are:

- I am okay and I am on my way.

- Acceptance is my answer for today.

- I grow through what I go through.

Upskill

Learn something new. Before undertaking the task of writing this book, I was studying psychology. Perhaps your schedule doesn't allow you to take on casual or part-time study; however, there are weekly classes you could attend, such as Clubbercise. Look it up: 1990s dance floor bangers, glow sticks and dancing in the dark — yes, Queen! There are DIY workshops, online short courses, instrument tutorials, paint by numbers activities, language classes, social card playing groups, working bees, arts and crafternoons. There may be subsidy kickbacks from your employer for upskilling at work. It's worth asking the question and finding something new and useful to do with all that spare time you now have. You'll feel like a superhero with your new skillset and a sense of achievement for setting out to complete something and doing it.

Do some breath work

If you find meditation a snooze fest, then this might be more for you. It's breathing, which we all do about 119 000 times a day without really thinking about it. Focused breath work is amazing, free and super easy. So you'll ace this! The benefits of breath work are so well publicised that it's becoming more mainstream. Some of the physical health benefits of breathwork may include balanced blood pressure, more time in deep sleep, a reduction of negative feelings, stronger respiratory function, an improved immune system and the release of stress hormones from your body.

Here is a basic guided breathing exercise.

Close your lips and use your nose to inhale slowly from your belly. Count to 4 as you breathe in, filling the lungs. Hold the air in your lungs while you silently count from 1 to 4, and then slowly release the air through your mouth as you count from 1 to 4. Repeat three to seven times.

Practise self-care

Add a splash of self-care into your day.

Here's a self-care menu:

- Go for a walk before everyone else wakes up.
- Practise some yoga.
- Do some breath work.
- Have a cold shower.
- Drink a cup of tea.
- Listen to a body-scan meditation.
- Go for a run.
- Book a massage.
- Run a bath. If you don't have a bath, get a bucket and dunk your feet in some Epsom salts.
- Pop some sugar in your coffee.
- Play some music.
- Have a nap.
- Sing out loud at the top of your lungs.
- Do a random act of kindness.
- Do something adventurous (waterslide, rollercoaster).
- Vacuum (a personal one that always helps me feel better).

Practise grounding

Grounding, or earthing, is also good for your soul. And it allows you to take off your shoes! The benefits of grounding include improved sleep, normalisation of the day–night cortisol rhythm, reduction in stress and a shift in the autonomic nervous system from sympathetic towards parasympathetic activation. Grounding techniques include walking barefoot in nature, on grass, dirt, farmland, sand or a nature track; lying on the ground; and submersing yourself in water. Sitting and placing your palms on the ground is also an easy way to access the benefits of grounding.

Do some handy work

Doing stuff with our hands feels good, and when you don't have a drink in your hand you might want to find something for your hands to do. Especially if one of your drinking places is on the couch watching TV. Take up knitting, sewing, painting, do some DIY, a puzzle, gardening — there are plenty of options and doing an activity with your hands will distract you from those thinking about drinking moments. There is beauty in creating something with our hands, whether it be a bread bin, an egg carton crocodile or some music. You can also search for a working bee in the local community or find a community garden that needs care.

Give back

You know the whole pay-it-forward philosophy — there's a movie about it. Oprah is hot on this, as am I. Doing something lovely for someone else can impact you positively. Whether it's volunteering at a shelter, dropping a meal on the neighbour's doorstep, getting involved in a charity, a local community event, being a car park coordinator at church, meals on wheels — there are so many areas in the community that can benefit from some extra help and a good attitude. I like to believe that sometimes it takes honouring someone else's vision for yours to shine too. Call it being a good Samaritan, a community caretaker, a friend to the friendless. Call it whatever you want — it works. Donate some clothes to an op-shop, give up your time for someone who is doing it tough, volunteer for a charity, mow your neighbour's lawn. There are endless possibilities and countless opportunities for you to be of service to others and you will feel so good.

Have a good laugh

Laughter is the best medicine and a great circuit-breaker. Find a comedy to watch, listen to a funny podcast, watch people injuring themselves on Instagram. Whatever you find funny, seek that out and laugh out loud. Laugh so hard you let a bit of wee out. Laugh until you cry. Laughter therapy may include laughter exercises, clowns, comedy movies, books, games and puzzles. It's also called humour therapy. It's a real thing! LOL!

Tune out

Keep your ears on, in a bid to block out the noise. Sometimes silence is the enemy. When that story in your head has become unhelpful, listening to a podcast, an audio book or some music can be a great distraction. I highly recommend my sober living podcast *Last Drinks* for inspiring stories about sobriety, but if you want to zone out and not think about sobriety for a bit, I totally get it. Sometimes a complete audible distraction can do wonders for your mindset.

Read

If you are a book nerd, which you might well be as you're reading this book, then stick your nose into a new book and if your schedule allows for it, read every day. Personally, I find a physical book is a better solution than scrolling the internet where pop-ups and distractions can appear. Taking yourself away to a quiet place and reading a book is nurturing, and you might learn something too. I love going to the library. It's peaceful (until some lady starts complaining loudly that the photocopier 'ate' her coins and isn't working). Overall, though, it is a great place to find some quiet time to just sit and read.

Write

Write a card, a letter, an email, a sticky note. Write something lovely and send it to someone. Write a letter of thanks, a note of appreciation, a compliment and give it to someone. Leave a note of love bombs in a lunchbox for someone to find, post a letter to a pen-pal. Get writing and you'll start to see the people you care about smile. Or write an entry of gratitude in your journal.

Talk

It's good to talk. Pick up the phone and call someone. A friend, a parent, a counsellor. Talking it out is helpful. Talking things through helps you to release tension, rather than keeping it inside. Talking about your feelings can help you stay in a healthy headspace and deal effectively with times when you feel troubled. It isn't a sign of weakness. It's part of taking charge of your wellbeing and doing what you can to stay healthy in your head.

Splash water

Sometimes just jumping into a body of water can completely transform you. If you live near the beach, then I suggest you get in that beautiful ocean to take your mind away. There is something resetting about the ocean. It's referred to in wellness as 'blue therapy'. Rich in magnesium, saltwater helps release stress, relax your muscles and promote deep sleep. Swimming in the ocean has also been linked to stimulating the parasympathetic system, which is responsible for rest and repair and can trigger the release of dopamine and serotonin. If you're not ocean side, then a lake, a river, a bath, a dam, the sprinkler or that trusty cold shower can act as an excellent supplement.

Get into the kitchen

Making something delicious to eat is a wholesome process. Food isn't meant to be delivered to our doorstep, ordered through an app, as convenient as this is. The process of finding a recipe, sourcing whole ingredients and taking the time to make something from scratch to either enjoy or share with others is a nurturing and nourishing process that you can learn to love. Become a MasterChef, a baker, a cake maker, a pie professional or a croquembouche conqueror.

Netflix and chill

Sometimes, just having a night in with a movie, a hot water bottle and a dairy-free ice-cream is good therapy. Learning to relax has taken me some time. In fact, I am still working on it. I find relaxing hard. Isn't that weird? It's not difficult to relax, but I am a doer, a go-getter. I am better under pressure. To just sit and enjoy a movie of an evening is something I am *learning* to enjoy. Letting go of the to-do list, the endless chores, hypothetical conversations and worst-case scenarios that can fly around in my brain at space ranger hyper speed, is a challenge. But I am trying, and I am improving, you'll be happy to hear. So, try to relax. I know there is nothing more annoying than someone telling you to relax, but try. The washing can wait, the people-pleasing can hit pause, the world won't end if you take five, 10 or 90 and relax. Do your best to try not to fall asleep on the couch; be present with what you are watching. Make it enjoyable, a simple pleasure. Then switch it off.

Activity: constructing your Sober Toolkit

Write out the top sober tools for your personal Sober Toolkit. Remember, you can refer to this as often as you need, and you can continue to curate this toolkit as you progress through sobriety.

Summing up ...

+ There are many wonderful benefits you will experience from a life without alcohol. Make some room in your journal to note them down as you experience them.

+ Find the strategies that speak to you and that will work for you and learn to lean into them. Do what works for you.

+ Writing a goodbye letter to alcohol will help you accept that a change is ahead.

+ Articulating one clear reason for your sobriety is important as it will reinforce your choice when you hit a tough spot — and there will be tough spots. But you can do this.

+ Setting up a connected sober support system is essential for your sober journey to help you and keep you safe and accountable during this time.

+ Nail down your sober response and learn it to avoid awkward conversations about your sobriety.

+ Adding in a goal for you to achieve throughout this experiment, aside from being sober, may act as a motivation for goal-orientated people.

(continued)

- Listing out some power moves you can lean into when you are in different environments is helpful. Preparing yourself for being in the world while being sober is important.

- Your personal Sober Toolkit is essential. You can continue to curate and refresh it throughout your sober journey. Fold in new tools that work for you. And then guess what? You are ready!

Part III

Your last drink

The best way to get started is to start. Before we hold hands and skip along the yellow brick road of sobriety success together, here's a heads up about what to expect from this next season as you engage in your daily routine without alcohol. I want you to *enjoy* this process. There will be some tough moments, some joy, and ultimately some growth and discovery. The truth is, this is not going to be easy — *sorry*, it's just not — and I can't pretend that it is. However, it is doable, and it is going to be worth it. Changing your behaviour is a process. It will involve your entire being and your complete attention. This is not to say it will hijack your entire day; you just need to commit to the work. Discovering your sober self won't necessarily *solve* all your problems, but what sobriety does, is afford you a clear head and a laser focus so you can navigate any situation fully present and from within your best, most balanced self. You are so brave for taking this step, for drawing a line in the sand to see what's on the other side of it. You are the only person who can rewrite your story. I hope you feel empowered and excited about what's to come. I am.

It won't be easy, but it will be worth it.

Time is our greatest commodity, which is why I was so clear on the intention of this book. I have written it from a place of compassion and experience. Remember, I had my 'day 1' too and I know how equally challenging and rewarding sobriety can be. By now you will have the tools you need to get started and you can continue to evolve your Sober Toolkit along the way.

I appreciate you for spending your valuable time reading this book. I understand you could have chosen to do so many other things with your time. Yet here we are. We have arrived at the business end. This is the action section. This is the start of your sobriety. If you have not had a drink today, then guess what? You are at day 1 of the 'Sober 30'. Go you!

The Sober 30

The Sober 30 — which is the topic of the remaining chapters of this book — is an exploration to uncover what will work for you instead of drinking — whether it's to relax, to cope, to celebrate or to decompress. It's a practical handbook for your first 30 days without alcohol that will help you to curate your own blueprint for what works in sobriety for you. So, pick out what you love and leave what doesn't rock your socks, float your boat or tickle your pickle.

All you need to do is commit to three things:

1. Read the daily Sober 30 reading.

2. Complete the daily Sober 30 activity.

3. Do not drink alcohol.

Some days will be a breather for you and other days you might feel flat or overwhelmed. When you have those off moments, go to your Sober Toolkit and grab one of the tools.

The early stages of this process can be a lot like starting out at the gym. Not the intimidating part — that is, when you're not sure where to look or how long to stretch for afterwards. Not that part. When you start working out, you go to the gym, work out and then you rest. The rest days let your muscles grow. Your muscles don't grow at the gym; they get torn apart at the gym and then they repair and grow during the rest period. Sobriety parallels to this philosophy. You start your sober journey, you stop drinking, then you need time and space to reflect and to adopt new strategies on how to spend your time and how to engage in your world without alcohol. In this time of repair, you will grow. And eventually, sobriety becomes effortless — your new normal. Just to confirm, this is about you discovering your sober self. Please be kind and show yourself compassion. Rest more, take baths, breathe deeply and commit to seeing this through, to finding out what is on the other side of your last drink.

The Sober 30 is a two-pillar approach founded in wholeness — your mind thinking positively, and your body working in a new way — that will result in your sober self being nurtured.

The combination of reading and doing each day will see you shift from going about your day on autopilot to living intentionally. Living without alcohol is challenging. You can feel strong in your choice for a couple of days but when the road gets bumpy, and autopilot is reactivated, you might want to reach for a drink to stop the thoughts that start circling in your mind. This is normal. Remember, you have been using alcohol as your coping mechanism for a while now. The thought of having a drink might come, but it will pass just as quickly if you can just sit with the thoughts and not engage with them. The daily activities are practical. They are designed to steer you out of your head and engage in something new. The activities are simple and fun. Some might be a bit weird, but just go with it. Embrace it all. The Sober 30 will give you some structure in your early sobriety. Remember, we thrive when we're in a routine, and this will become the glue behind your sobriety.

Read, do, rest.

Repeat.

7 Setting up for the Sober 30

In preparation for the Sober 30, please do the following:

- Throw out any alcohol in your house.

   Why? Because I don't trust you! Nah, I'm kidding. I totally trust you, but having a bottle of vino in the fridge is only going to tempt you on day 12 when you feel mentally strong but you think, *Well, one glass wouldn't hurt.* Take the temptation away. You have a 100 per cent better chance of sticking to your Sober 30 with 0 per cent alcohol in the house. It's that simple. If it's not in the house, you can't drink it.

- Tell a trusted friend.

   This does *not* include updating your Facebook status, tweeting it or posting an 'Alcohol-Free Zone' sign on your Insta story. Just find one or two of your nearest and dearest who you can ask for support and to whom you can be accountable. Being honest with someone you trust can be a relief during this process. Find a trusted friend, or talk to your mum (or someone else's). Remember, the people who matter don't see you as you see yourself, so let the right person be your rock.

- Complete the daily activities with a smile.

  This is the plan I curated when I went from alcohol at everything to totally sober. It worked for me, and I feel like you and I are cut from the same cloth, you know? I used the first month away from alcohol to try out a whole bunch of new stuff I had always wanted to. I looked at the month like a crazy adventure, full of new things I'd always wanted to try. So, knock yourself out trying new things and enjoying new experiences.

- Write in your journal each day.

  Start or end each day with an entry in your journal. It may just be one thing you are grateful for, what you are looking forward to, an intention, a gripe, what's coming up for you or what's challenging for you. Journalling helps in the organisation of thoughts and feelings.

Over the next month, you'll become awakened to your thoughts, your feelings, your own truth and to so many things you might have missed had you carried on carrying on every weekend/week/day/waking moment. This isn't about feeling bad for past choices; it's about feeling empowered for the work you are doing in the present, in making *you* more connected with your best and sober self here, now, today. The Sober 30 is a gentle nudge in a new direction, offering some structure and a rhythm. Once the 30 days are done, my advice is to keep going, keep exploring and accessing your Sober Toolkit. A full season of sobriety will give you a deeper understanding of what your best life looks like because you will see it take shape.

Congratulations for choosing to march forward into the discovery of your own personal truth. The reward will come. The fruits of your labour *will* be harvested. For now, your focus is clear. You have decided to put *you* first. You have had your last drink.

*A **disclaimer:** You may want to consult your GP before having your last drink because the physical side-effects for heavy drinkers may be dangerous. The guidance of a doctor and/or a trained therapist is my highest recommendation when changing your lifestyle — and I am not a doctor, nor a therapist.*

*A **quiet side note:** If you do slip up, please be kind to yourself, acknowledge the slip-up and start again. Use this as an opportunity to become aware of the trigger and try again. Keep going.*

Ready? Okay!

8 30 benefits in 30 days

When I stopped drinking, I suddenly, *accidentally*, started kicking life in the literal pants. My single, sober decision led to open doors, opportunities, paradigm shifts and 'aha' moments. Sure, there were some super tough moments in there too. Over time, I noticed good things coming my way. By choosing to spend my time doing anything other than what 95 per cent of grown adults do on a weekend (not an actual statistic, more of a guesstimate), I allowed my head some space to create a new narrative. I spent quality time reading and learning. I rewarded myself with compassion, which flowed to other areas of my life. It was a ripple effect.

One small decision every day led to bigger and more beautiful things down the track.

Peace, it does not mean to be in a place where there is no noise, trouble, or hard work. It means to be in the midst of those things and still be calm in your heart.
Unknown

The overwhelming benefits of sobriety can be found splashed across 'quit drinking' websites, blogs, personal stories in the news, #soberliving #alcoholfree movements, foundations and communities. It is our shared experiences that are most powerful. Here are 30 benefits you can brace yourself for:

1. *You will experience the sheer joy of waking up sober repeatedly.* This feels so good, and it won't get boring. Waking up refreshed will eventually overshadow any desire to stay out late, because waking up fresh, energised and with a smile is the best.

2. *Your liver will begin to rejuvenate.* This doesn't seem like a sexy benefit, but your liver function is important. Although this is an 'inside' benefit, the liver plays a central role in all metabolic processes in the body. It breaks down fats to produce energy. So you'll have more energy.

3. *Your hair and nails will strengthen.* I hear the blokes sigh, 'Great, that's awesome Maz', but your hair and nail strength is a direct reflection of your immune system strength. So you'll be stronger.

4. *You will be rich.* You will save so much cash — not that anyone uses cash anymore — so there'll be some extra fat in your piggy bank this month.

5. *Your brain will begin to heal.* That 'foggy' feeling in your brain will, slowly but surely, lift. It will take a little bit of time but soon enough that wonderful feeling of being able to think clearly and deeply will return.

6. *You will sleep so well.* Your body doesn't need to detox poison so your circadian rhythm returns, and you will sleep better.

7. *There will be no more sneaking around.* I used to underestimate how many drinks I'd had because the real number sounded bad, and I would always feel guilty about this. You too? Oh, glad it wasn't just me. Well, you won't have the drink guilts anymore.

8. *You'll be glowing gorgeous.* Your skin will improve, redness will disappear, dark circles will lift — you're going to look great. Alcohol dehydrates you, depleting you of nutrients, which shows up on your face. Watch this space ... rather, watch your face!

9. *You'll just feel better.* It only takes a couple of days and you'll feel better about yourself, about life in general — damn, you'll feel so good!

10. *You'll have so much more free time.* You used to spend a lot of time just hanging out at a bar talking nonsense, but these days you'll finally have some extra time to learn a language, start cross stitching, take up a social sport, study that course you've always talked about, read a book ... or write a book!

11. *Wait, is it compliments week?* It sure is. Family, friends, co-workers: they'll all notice a new spring in your step, and they'll feel compelled to tell you or even ask you what your secret is.

12. *Is this* The Matrix? You'll have this new way of seeing things: you'll notice the birds singing, the sun on your face, the little things. A fresh soda water with some lime in it will feel like angel tears on your tongue.

13. *You'll have a new bestie!* You'll start to like yourself again. You might not have thought about it much, but would you want to hang out with you? Well, you will now, because you are a sober, empowered, wonderful person.

14. *You'll not just be a goal setter, you'll be a goal smasher.* Setting a personal goal to live alcohol free is a big deal, and completing that task is an even bigger deal. Being able to set a goal, and stay true to it, empowers you.

15. *You'll have positive vibes only.* As you begin to feel stronger and healthier, you will have a renewed sense of optimism for the days ahead of you.

16. *You'll see your friendships for what they represent.* And perhaps you'll be emboldened to do some friendship-garden pruning, which is perfect. If you want to fly with eagles, surround yourself with eagles.

17. *Hello Einstein! You'll feel like a creative genius.* It's like an actual lightbulb flicked on inside your head. No more coming up with great ideas that end up in the gutter. Fresh ideas will be flowing.

18. *Did you just become a scientist?* Probably not, unless you *are* a scientist; in which case, can you please explain why we still tie up our shoes with shoelaces? Anyway, whether you are or aren't a scientist, you'll feel like experimenting — you'll feel more adventurous.

19. *You won't make any more stupid decisions* (or if you do make a stupid decision, you'll at least be 100 per cent aware that you are making a stupid decision).

20. *You'll be nicer, less angry and have more patience.*

21. *You'll smell good.* No more next day reek of booze. You'll smell as fresh as a flower in a flowerpot.

22. *You'll significantly reduce your risk of cancer.*

23. *Rather than being on the sauce, you'll become the source.* If you still go out with your friends — and you can — you'll become a reliable source of information. Suddenly, your credibility is through the roof, and all you did was stay sober.

24. *No more trying to figure out what happened last night.* Your memory will be on point.

25. *Have you lost weight?* Quite possibly, a side-effect of consuming fewer empty calories, for some, is a slight slimming down. In fact, cutting out alcohol for a month can result in weight loss of between 2 and 4 kilograms.

26. *You'll have empathy overload.* You may find you are more sensitive to others' needs and have more empathy and compassion. As you start to get to know your sober self better, you'll develop a bigger capacity for those around you.

27. *You'll have exploration overload.* You'll have so much time to do new things, try new ways to relax and fill up your day.

28. *You'll be more focused, and your productivity will increase — and maybe even your reproductivity.* You will be able to concentrate more and be less flighty with your thoughts.

29. *You'll be putting your health first by choosing sobriety.* This level of self-care is infectious.

30. *You'll be your better self.* And you'll be showing up and doing life fully present to the power of rad.

You are wonderful.

You are ready.

You've got this.

•••

In the chapters that follow, we'll look at each day of the Sober 30 in more detail.

Day 1

Good morning sunshine. Welcome. I'm so glad you're here. Today you are taking the very first step on your new alcohol-free journey. Here we go.

Today might be a breeze, or it might be bloody awful, but either way, the great thing is that no matter what happens — whether you finally see a unicorn, win an endless supply of paperclips or find where all the missing socks ended up — you *are* going alcohol free. It's a simple choice. *Even if* you meet your childhood idol, or something terrible happens like the world runs out of coconut yoghurt, today is the first day that you won't be swigging some Savvy B or splashing some Kahlua on your Coco Pops.[3] There are one billion different scenarios that could play out today, which is super exciting, or slightly anxiety inducing, depending on your personality type. The best news is that you already have set an intention for the day, regardless of any curve ball thrown your way.

Today I am sober.

Today I honour my choice to live without alcohol.

Today is a good day.

Your life experience is the sum of your choices. Change your decisions and you will change your life. If nothing changes, *nothing*

---

[3] I did this once on a snowboarding trip in early 2000 at Perisher. I also broke my wrist that day.

changes, but today is about making one simple change. Sobriety is about coming to each moment with the innate trust in your own ability to wander through the world today, without a drink. And you are so capable. Now, if you find yourself facing a difficult situation and reaching for the Rosé, which has been your default behaviour in the past, *today* you can look through a new lens. You can choose differently. Actively, consciously. Make a new choice today that will honour your sober self. Regardless of the day of the week or the type of underwear you have on, I know you can get through today without a drink. So, get on with it my friend! The day is waiting.

Today's activity

Write down three things you are grateful for and three things you like about yourself in your journal. Oh, and before I forget, take a few selfies. No filter, regular lighting. We will circle back to these photos in about a month.

Day 2

Two. That's the magic number. No wait, sorry, that's three. My apologies. I'm getting ahead of myself. It's day 2. This is huge. You have successfully navigated a full 24 hours without a drink. You got through the first day. Let's get through the next. On a physical level, your liver is doing a great job of processing the toxins of alcohol out of your blood stream. It's not fully done, but it's getting there. Your liver is the organ responsible for removing alcohol from your body, so you are still most likely in a detox phase. Give it some time. Let your body do its thing. And remember to drink plenty of water.

How good is not being hungover? Hangover-free mornings are the best.

The first week without alcohol will let your body recalibrate to its natural baseline and give your brain some time to catch up to what's going on. The new choice to *not drink* is a new thought process for your brain to wrap itself around. Be prepared for your body to do some funky stuff. You might feel tired, you may have a headache, your number twos might be a brand-new experience as the toxins start to dislodge from your previous alcohol consumption, even though it was *only two glasses*.[4] You don't have to write a tell-all memoir about it today. Just stick to the plan, drink lots of water and rest up. Give your body and brain the space they need to get used to this new way of living.

---

[4]We all know that is code for a bottle. It's okay. I said it too.

Some symptoms and some sweet relief:

- *Headaches*: Rub a drop of rosemary essential oil on your temples in a light circular motion or pop a couple of drops of chamomile essential oil in a dehumidifier next to your bed. You can make a DIY room spray using filtered water, lavender essential oil and a spray bottle.

- *Dehydration*: Drink room temperature water with a fresh squeeze of lemon. Drink consistently throughout the day. Water is your new drink of choice. Hydrating foods like cucumber, radishes, celery, cabbage and watermelon can make for a good hydrating lunch choice.

- *Tiredness*: A cold shower will wake you up. Or you can go for a brisk walk in the fresh air or take a power nap for 20 minutes.

- *Crankiness*: Go for a walk, or try a 10-minute breathing exercise. Stay offline.

- *Sugar craving*: Fresh berries and Greek yoghurt will do the trick. Eat a banana, or smash a *big* tablespoon of peanut butter or an apple dipped in almond butter.

If you *think* about having a drink, *decide* not to. It's a mind hack. Now you know you have the choice, you can make the choice! If something annoying happens, like your car breaks down, you drop your entire coffee on the ground or find some new greys in your hair, remember *that a drink won't change what has already happened*, so you can easily stick with your decision to be alcohol free.

Today's activity

Enjoy a few minutes of mindfulness. If you already have a mindfulness practice, then go for it. There are loads of mindfulness and meditation apps available. See the section 'Your Sober Toolkit' at the back of the book for a list of my recommendations.

When I am feeling anxious or overwhelmed, or I'm unable to fall asleep, I complete the following 4, 7, 8 breathing technique.

Find a quiet space and sit comfortably, or you can lie down.

Close your eyes.

Breathe in through your nose for four counts, hold your breath in for seven counts and then breathe out through your mouth for eight counts.

4

7

8

This is one round.

Repeat this breathing rhythm for *four rounds*.

Congratulations. You've completed a few minutes of mindfulness.

Day 3

Think about all the sweet cash you are going to start saving by not buying alcohol! Think of all the rounds of drinks you won't be shouting your friends at the pub, or the bottles of wine with dinner you won't be sipping casually, or Espresso Martinis with dessert you won't be ordering. Over the next few weeks there will be plenty of situations that would require you to buy alcohol and splash out on some booze. Going alcohol free changes the maths equation. In my first year in sobriety, I estimated a saving of more than $10 000. Here is the skinny on my savings.

Average spends:

- A bottle of wine with dinner a few times a week ($30) (×3) (×52 weeks)

- Presents for birthdays each month, a good bottle of champagne ($80) (×12)

- One big night out on the town ($100) (×52 weeks) not including a taxi home or dry cleaning.

Q: How much money did I save in one year by giving up alcohol?
A: $(3 \times \$30 \times 52) + (\$80 \times 12) + (\$100 \times 52)$
$= 4680 + 960 + 5200 = \$10\,840$

At the end of the year, I went on a holiday to Thailand for 10 days and drank from coconuts and rode a scooter in my bikini. Do your own equation. Figure out how much money you are saving over the 30 days and then see what that equates to over a year. It's quite motivating, don't you think?

Today's activity

Start a piggy bank. You can go and get an actual pig piggy bank, you can recycle a coconut oil jar or you can just open a separate savings account. Just find somewhere to put your savings and any time you would have spent money on alcohol, save those dollars in the piggy bank. And then have a think about how you want to spend your savings.

Day 4

Look at you, you're bravely trying out a new way of living. That's huge. Give yourself a high five, and as you do, say 'self-five' out loud. You may have found the last few days were a walk in the park, or they may have been your most challenging ever. Either way, you're doing great! Keep going.

What soap is for the body, tears are for the soul.
Jewish Proverb

Now that you're not smashing cans or sipping champers, you're most likely feeling some emotions. I'm not sure of the science on this, but most people I have spoken to who have stopped drinking admit that within the first few days, some big feelings start to surface. Let those feelings out! There are lots of ways you can handle this, despite it being uncomfortable. You can just cry if crying is your thing. It might be helpful to confide in a friend, or do some exercise to get those endorphins pumping. You might want to write in your journal, or just sit and sob. If you are letting the feelings flow, you are making progress. And it's totally okay. Cry ... maybe not on the bus. But hey, if it hits you on the B-line go with it; allow yourself to *feel* again. Emotions are not logical, but they *are* very real. I guess in some ways I am similar. I am a very real person with a lack of logic at times!

As your body begins to reprogram its baseline, clarity returns and your emotions will kick into gear again. The past habit of suppressing your emotions, or at least stifling them, was keeping your feelings away, but now you can begin to process them as they come up. You have the space you need to begin to sort out some of your stuff. And we all have stuff. Emotional stuff requires strength in the form of vulnerability. Your emotions might seem to just simmer under the radar and then suddenly jump out and karate chop you in the face. Take some tissues with you and excuse yourself from the board meeting if you must.

Today's activity

Go for a walk through nature today for an hour if you can — or at least for 20 minutes. Don't take any technology. Just listen to your surroundings and your heart, and don't get lost. And buy a few boxes of tissues on your way home.

Day 5

Good morning! And how do you feel today? Not hungover? Excellent. Get used to that. You're on your way to more of these pleasant morning experiences.

Here is the good news:

Your biggest physical alcohol detox hurdle is well and truly over. It takes about 48 hours for your body to rid itself of *all* the alcohol in your system, depending on how many weekends away in wine country you've attended. It may have taken a few extra hours for some. Now your body is through the detox phase! Yay. How are those emotions going?

Let's talk about the threshold of excellence: it's one of my rules for life. It's doing the very best to be excellent in any situation, even the average ones. It's part of what led to my alcohol relationship reassessment. I realised when I drank, my standards dropped: the act of drinking led me to be a bit of an idiot. Not a monster, but not an excellent person either. If I wanted the 'threshold of excellence' to be upheld in every area of my life — through every hurdle, heartbreak and kick-ass moment — then I needed an alcohol reframe because my behaviour was bringing down the threshold.

The threshold of excellence is a state of mind that infiltrates your *whole* approach to life.

Today's activity

Find an affirmation that you can fold into your self-talk. And whenever you think about it, say it to yourself. Write it down and stick it on your bathroom mirror, on your laptop screen or on your iPhone wallpaper so you will see it constantly throughout the day and continually be saying something affirming to yourself. Here are three of my personal favourites. These will help redesign the self-talk in your head and help wire new neurons of positivity and sobriety together.

1. I am braver than I think, stronger than I know and more loved than I can ever imagine.

2. All I need is within me right now.

3. I always get to where I'm going by walking away from where I have been. (Yes, this is from *Winnie the Pooh*, and I love it.)

Day 6

Wrap your head around the fact that this is an *empowering* choice, not a punishment because you were 'out of control'. Please don't feel bad that you might miss out on a party or two over the next weekend or so. Feel excited that there is a whole new part of the day you're experiencing. As best you can, just do one moment at a time, one day at a time, for the bigger-than-you reason that you articulated in the Sober Synopsis activity in chapter 6. And if you are feeling guilt over the past, you can leave that backpack at the door. Guilt can be crippling, but that's completely unhelpful. It's a redundant emotion. Guilt occurs when we believe or realise, whether it be accurate or not, that we have compromised our standards of conduct. Drinking, at the core of it, is one big compromise of our personal standards. So, the guilt may be real for you right now as you spend time reflecting on days gone by. However, rather than sit in the negativity that can come with feelings of guilt, you can use this emotion to help acknowledge your actions and fuel your motivation to stay sober and improve your behaviour. Every emotion serves a purpose and when we allow ourselves to experience guilty feelings as a way of receiving information, we are already healing from our mistakes. Guilt lets us know that our actions conflict with our values and can help us to repair the damage.

Today's activity

Now that we have tackled some emotional stuff, let's eat! Get yourself into the kitchen and make some protein balls with a hint of natural sugar to get you through those sugar cravings. Here are two of my fave recipes.

You're welcome.

Lemon Coconut Balls

Ingredients

3/4 cup cashews

1/3 cup desiccated coconut

1 tbs chia seeds

2 tbs rice malt syrup or agave nectar

1/2 tsp vanilla extract

2 tbs water

2 tbs fresh lemon juice

Method

Place the cashews in a food processor to form a crumbly cashew mixture.

Transfer the cashew mixture to a bowl. Add the coconut, chia seeds, rice malt syrup, vanilla extract, water and lemon juice and combine (add more water if required). Divide the mixture into five piles and roll each pile into a ball in the palm of your hands. Set in the fridge for half an hour.

1 ball = 1 serve

Chocolate Salty Balls

Ingredients

1 cup almonds

3 or 4 tbs raw cacao + extra to roll the balls in

1 tbs coconut sugar + extra to roll the balls in

1/2 tsp vanilla extract

8 or 9 dates

1 tbs coconut oil

pinch sea salt

Method

Mix all the ingredients in a food processor. Roll into balls and then roll in the extra cacao and coconut sugar. Refrigerate for half an hour. Enjoy!

Day 7

Hey superstar! Think about what was going on a week ago. You hadn't *not* had a drink for a whole week, that's for sure. In the past seven days, you have hopefully had 56 hours of sleep, eaten 3.5 cups of oats for breakfast — if oats are your thing — ordered eight takeaway coffees (assuming you have two on a Saturday like any regular person), hit the gutter while reverse parking once (maybe twice) and consumed zero alcoholic drinks. What a week!

> *It probably comes as no surprise that there's a very perceptible improvement in both physical and mental health when you stop drinking. Aside from the obvious absence of any hangover, physically I felt better rested, more energetic and was able to hit 'personal bests' both in the gym and during cardiovascular exercise. Physical exercise fuels the production of serotonin and dopamine, which leads to an elevated mood, leading to a positive feedback loop to want to continue exercising (and, of course, the release of the feelgood brain chemicals also leads to a boost in overall mental health). Mentally, again, no hangovers so no 'hangxiety'. Much more clarity throughout the day, and an overall improvement in mood and general wellbeing because of no longer introducing a depressant into my system. These improvements (both physical and mental) start slowly but compound quickly over time.*
> **Dr Matt Agnew — science communicator and author**

In your physical body, after a week of not binge drinking, things are starting to normalise and your sugar cravings are possibly through the roof. Try to stick to a piece of fruit for a sugar hit or have those protein balls you made yesterday on standby. Oh look, if you *really* must, do as I do and invest in a Twix. Truly the best and most perfect chocolate bar on the planet! Oh, the crumbling crunch of the biscuit base, perfectly complementing the ooze of the sweet sugary caramel that explodes through the chocolate hug it's cradled in. I have spent a *lot* of time thinking about how awesome a Twix is. The bottom line is, you are starting to feel the positive impacts of no alcohol both physically and mentally. The benefits are starting to showcase. Sobriety is looking good on you. Again, if you feel a craving for alcohol, remind yourself it will pass and refer to your Sober Toolkit if you need to.

Today's activity

Reflect in your journal how you felt one week ago, the day before you began this quest, and compare it to how you are feeling now. You can talk about your physical feelings, your mental health, your opinion of yourself and notice if anything has started to shift or come up for you. This journal entry is observational and about awareness. There is no word count limitation. Just write until you feel done. And find a new way to celebrate a milestone. Have a look in your Sober Toolkit to see if something jumps out at you that you can try out to mark the one-week milestone of sobriety. Go celebrate one week of sobriety!

Day 8

One of the keys in forming healthy and new habits is to focus your attention on what to do or what you have rather than spiral around what you are stopping or going without. When I became a vegetarian, as short lived as it was, rather than look at a menu at a café and read through all the options that I genuinely wanted but wasn't allowing myself—like the BLAT, the bacon and egg roll, or the pancakes with maple syrup and bacon (it was bacon that was my undoing as a makeshift vegetarian)—I would grab the menu and just flick to the vegetarian options. I would focus on what I could have, not what I was going without. In this season it is natural to use language like, 'I'm quitting alcohol' or 'I'm not drinking' and as much as these statements are true, the words have a negative inflection. Changing your dialogue around what you are doing will help it settle in your mind. Instead of looking at the next few weeks as something you will suffer through, let's reframe it into an exploration, a positive experience, an adventure, an opportunity. Move your thinking from what you are *not* doing by flipping the script and embracing positively charged words to articulate what's going on for you.

I'm choosing sobriety.

I'm taking a break from drinking.

I'll have a mineral water, thanks babe.

These three statements express your intention in a positive way. Interrupting old patterns of language takes an effort, but before long, like anything we repeat enough, it will become second nature and the more you do it the easier it gets. Even just repeating these positive sentences to yourself will start to create new neural pathways. The simple awareness of how you are speaking about yourself, and to yourself, is great progress.

Today's activity

Playtime. Find something fun to do that a little kid would choose to do. As adults, we simply forget to have fun, so have some fun today! Play! Jump on a trampoline, swim in the nude, climb a tree, dig in the sand, blow bubbles, make a mud pie, get dirty, make a slip n slide, play in a sprinkler, pick some flowers, run down the street with bare feet, dance in the lounge room, colour in, play with some playdough, knock and run, water fight, kick a footy, roll down a grass hill, lick the spoon, hopscotch, have a chalk chase or a scavenger hunt, skateboard, roller-skate, rollerblade, ride your bike, build a rocket, build a pillow fort, or have a pillow fight or a sock wrestle.

Day 9

You have most likely been guzzling a truckload of H2O in the past week or so. As well you should. Water is amazing stuff. Remember how your parents nagged you all the time about drinking eight glasses of water a day? Well, it turns out parents are usually right. Water does more than just quench your thirst and regulate your body's temperature; it also keeps the tissues in your body supple and helps retain optimum levels of moisture in the blood, bones and brain. Water also helps protect the spinal cord, and it acts as a lubricant and cushion for your joints. It can even make you smarter! The brain and heart are composed of 73 per cent water, and the lungs are about 83 per cent water. Your skin contains 64 per cent water; muscles and kidneys are 79 per cent water; and even your bones are watery — that's bones, not boners. It makes sense that we need to top up our tanks constantly with the fresh, slippery stuff so we can function. If you're wondering how much water you should drink, it's a totally individualised business. You can speak with your doctor for clarification if you are unsure. As a general rule, men should drink about 10 cups of water a day and women about eight cups.

Today's activity

Spend some time in a body of water today and or/buy a soda stream (#notsponsored). Have a bath. Go for an ocean swim, to the local pool, a water slide... whatever. Find a waterfall, a nature pool, a natural spring, a lake, a river. Take the family to a leisure centre. Spend some quality time in the wet stuff and enjoy it. You might find it works for you as part of your self-care. Take time out in some water *today*. And, by the way, a soda stream makes any glass of water fun. I'd be lost without mine.

Day 10

Ten days. Zero drinks. Wonderful. Here's a quick question for you: Have you heard of a 'de-lank'? De-lank is a word my husband and I legit invented. Its evolution came from a simple question one day: 'Are you cranky?' I'll let you guess who asked whom this loaded question. After a super-fun, non-passive-aggressive exchange of words, the conversation continued with, 'Hey cranks', which turned into 'crank-de-lank', which landed us at 'de-lank'. Now if either of us is a bit down in the dumps for a legitimate reason, or no reason at all, we affectionately refer to that person as 'de-lank'. It's a productive little hack that usually gets said person out of a funk, or at least talking about it so they can feel better. Now that you are not watering down emotions with some watered-down scotch, you're most likely *feeling* your emotions. Perhaps the lack of social lubricant has opened you up to some feelings you're not used to. In fact, you may feel a bit lightheaded, which for you right now feels weird, but that feeling is *clarity*. This is all new territory and it's completely okay to feel out of sorts. It's okay to feel a bit 'de-lank'. Just try not to simmer in it. Acknowledge you are feeling a bit flat and then do something that makes you feel better. You can go and pick a tool from your Sober Toolkit and do that thing that makes you feel good, and if you are stuck for a 'feel good because I'm not feeling good about my feelings' moment, here are my top five tools (I make them physical: as your body moves, your brain grooves):

1. Dance on the spot for two minutes.

2. Go for a 10-minute brisk walk.

3. Do a beautiful puppy pose yoga stretch.

4. Get upside down somewhere: a headstand, a handstand.

5. 5 × high kicks, 5 × spins, 5 × butt slaps (on your own butt).

Or you can buy a puppy! No — too far. Sorry I took it too far. Remember to take some time out when you're feeling overloaded. If today is one of those days, you might feel tempted to drink because that has been your go-to response. If you're in a bit of a funk and feeling like a sooky pants, don't dive for the bottle — try a new way of getting yourself out of grinch mode.

Today's activity

Today is worth celebrating. You are worth celebrating. You are doing so well. If only two good things happened today, you may as well take the wins and celebrate 10 days of being sober. You have made a commitment to your future self and remained faithful to that decision. And that means you are finally putting *you first*. And that means you are well on your way to becoming the best version of you ever. And that, my friend, is certainly worth celebrating (fist pump). Celebrating doesn't always have to involve spending, but hey, you're only human, and retail therapy has its pluses.

Here are my 'celebrate you' suggestions. Pick one and try it out:

+ Splurge on dessert.

+ Go to that brunch place on everyone's Instagram feed.

+ Buy those shoes.

+ Organise a games night with friends.

+ Buy new pjs.

(*continued*)

- Book that fancy dinner.

- Get your hair/nails done.

- Schedule a massage.

- Cash in that Groupon voucher your distant cousin gave you for Christmas, and do the pizza-making class or stand-up paddle boarding adventure.

- Have one sugar in your coffee — hell, have two.

- Buy yourself some fresh flowers. Roses are perfect.

- Order in.

- Treat yourself to the movies and sit in the fancy seats.

- Buy an expensive candle and light it.

- Buy a puppy! Or puppy-sit if buying a puppy isn't really a viable option.

Day 11

11:11

Whenever I see the time at 11:11, I smile. I wasn't 100 per cent sure if 11:11 was a thing — or 111 per cent sure to be exact — so I did some research (which is code for googled it). And here is what I found: a lot of TikTok videos and a lot of noise about how special seeing the clock at 11:11 is. Not a lot of scientifically backed research, but enough of a vibe for me to include it today for you.

Now, I'm not huge on numerology. The only numbers I identify with are when something is on sale, but according to numerology a sequence of 1s means whatever you are thinking about is in the process of becoming. Think of it as the universe's way of helping us to pay attention to our heart, and our intuition. So that's encouraging. And now that I have put this on your radar, I bet you'll see it all the time. And when you do, I hope you feel good. It's like when you want to buy a yellow car and then, suddenly, every car you see on the road is yellow. It's weird, right? Well, this may be the case for you and the number 1, and I hope it makes you smile.

Today's activity

Go for a walk today for an hour — or an hour and 11 minutes — but don't listen to my podcast, *Last Drinks*, or anything else. Just listen to your surroundings, the sound of your breath, the

(continued)

tread of your steps, the crunch of the ground, the squeak of your knees, the swing of your arms, the thoughts in your head, the chafe of your thighs.

Just walk.

If walking isn't your thing, then do what works for you. A run, a bike ride, a kayak. Take some time out for yourself and get into some nature. Do something physical.

Day 12

If you are making a choice that is better for you and you have people around you who aren't on board with your journey, you need to reassess their position in your life. I found myself with the opportunity to meet new people who were supporting my choices because I was curating a new life. Your vibe attracts your tribe. You will attract the right people and the right opportunities to support your sobriety.
Action Alexa — motivation/fitness expert

Proximity is power. The people you have in your proximity need to be on your level. Let's talk about your friends, your mates, your buddies, your tribe, the crew. Not your Facebook friends or Instagram followers. I mean your human friends who know the true you. There are friends and followers who watch your online profile updates and interact with you with an emoji or occasional witty comment. Then there are the friends you engage with in life through shared experiences. Not to say that your real friends can't also be your online friends, but the number of people you call your true friends wouldn't be in the hundreds or tens of thousands. My friendship circle got tighter in sobriety. This was an invisible benefit and completely unintentional. The friendships that were solely fuelled by alcohol-filled nights seemed to dissipate quite naturally. At first I felt guilty, but soon enough I realised it's okay to let go. Letting go of people and things that didn't serve me or support my decision was okay.

You might be in a similar situation, and it is tough. But this process is about curating a scaffold of people in your life who serve you, encourage you and can accept you as you are: sober and thriving. As I spent more time in sobriety, the social invites did slow down. For me personally, this was a relief. I hadn't realised until sobriety that I am an extroverted introvert. Which means, I refuel by being at home. I just happen to have a big personality. So, when things dried up in my social diary, I was thrilled. I felt free. I was so happy to not have to battle the social anxiety being a true introvert offers. However, if you're an extrovert, this is going to be tough for you, and I feel for you. As an extrovert, you are refuelling by spending time with others, and that can be tricky if you are navigating sobriety. Sobriety and socialising can be a difficult match at first. This is where a new thing can be your lifeline. Socialising in situations that do not need alcohol can be your new way to refuel. If you can, find a new social group you can hang out with that doesn't involve booze. For example, a social tennis group, a walking group, the gym, squash, touch footy, a community garden, meals on wheels, a part-time job, a dance class, pottery, yoga or golf. Something where you can get your social fix without the pressure of alcohol. Perhaps your decision

You will find other people who are reassessing their relationship with alcohol will gravitate to you and start to pop up in your world.

to grow has been received as a minor threat to some people in your circles, and as the common link of tipples has dried up, there is no common ground for the friendship. You may find you let go of some people, or they may let go of you — and that's okay. This process is teaching you to be fluid, let go and respond well. You can't control others, only yourself.

'Show me your friends and I'll show you your future' — I do love a good Japanese proverb. Right now, you are experiencing a major self-reassessment and figuring yourself out. You will find other people who are reassessing their relationship with alcohol will gravitate to you and start to pop up in your world. The universe honours great decisions and aligns like-minded people alongside each other for encouragement so you can feel seen and heard. All you need sometimes is to know that someone else has walked the path and is willing to walk it alongside you.

Today's activity

Take some time to reflect on your friendships and assess how supportive your mates have been of your decision. Write about your friends in your journal:

+ Are they fully supportive of your decision and on the journey with you?

+ Have they dropped off the radar?

+ Are they just waiting for you to fail?

+ Have they managed to look at their own drinking behaviours?

The list of people who are closest to you — who you want to share your life with — are the contents of your friendship garden and I hope that yours is in great condition. If not, you may have some pruning to do. It's okay if your friendship garden is full, but after this exercise there may be some more room.

And sign up to a social group so you can engage with people where alcohol isn't on the table.

Day 13

You have so much clarity in sobriety. When you stop drinking, you start to get a new level of realisation of your own actions, who you are and healing.
Bex Weller — founder, Sexy Sobriety

In almost two weeks, your taste buds can taste again, and you can stop and smell the roses because:

- you have more time on your hands

- your senses are coming back, and you can *literally* smell the roses

- you (may have) bought yourself roses three days ago.

You are becoming an epically grounded, sober human. You may have experienced an intense level of FOMO (that's 'Fear of Missing Out', for Baby Boomers reading this). Maybe there was a last-minute invitation, or something that's been in the diary for months. Maybe you felt like going or maybe you stayed at home. With cases of FOMO, a quick re-framing can give you a lift. Instead of sitting at home being bummed out that you're not at the pub/club/bar/hotel/motel/Holiday Inn, think about the beautiful sunrise you're going to see tomorrow. That's right, tomorrow we are waking up at the crack of it, to welcome in the new day.

But that's tomorrow. Let's quickly talk about everyone else. You're good. You're nailing sobriety. Other people though? Upon reflection of your friendships, it may appear you don't have so much in common with some of the people you are used to kicking around with, apart from drinking. And when you take the drinks off the table, what else is there? You can totally still be buddies with your buddies, but it could be time to redefine some of those relationships to suit the boundaries you have placed around your habits. You are tapping into a whole new way to experience life. It's a bit *Matrix* isn't it, Neo? You are not missing out on anything you haven't *already* seen or heard before. So have a think about how you can redefine some of your relationships if they are worthy of your time. Brunch instead of bars, walks instead of whiskey, volunteering instead of vino, afternoon tea instead of afternoon tipples. Sober hangs are the fabric of sobriety.

Today's activity

Now, set your alarm for *before sunrise* tomorrow. You are waking up super early so you can see the beauty of the start of a new day. The best way to prepare for an early start (trust me, I host breakfast radio) is to set your alarm for the exact time you need to get up, not earlier so you can snooze. Do not give yourself a snooze option. When that alarm goes off, get straight out of bed.

How to get out of bed at a radically early time

As soon as your alarm sounds, immediately stand up, raise your hands in the air and walk out of your bedroom. Find the kitchen like a zombie and drink a glass of water. Take a deep breath in and out, and voilà. Good morning! *Do not snooze.* You snooze, you lose, don't even think about it. Just get up and out of bed before your brain knows what happening. Personally, I jump straight into a cold shower at 4 am. It's part

(continued)

of my morning routine. Yes, my alarm is set for 4 am weekdays. I get up, do 20 minutes of yoga and then have a cold shower. I am the perkiest 4 am waker-upperer there is! (Perkiness is optional.)

Another tactic: when your alarm goes off, say out loud '5, 4, 3, 2, 1 *blast off*' and when you say 'blast off', stand up. This might be annoying for the other person in your bed if there is one, so use with caution.

Day 14

Rise and shine wonderful human! Did you snooze? I hope not. With any luck you managed to get yourself out of bed when the alarm went off and you haven't fallen back to sleep in the corner of your kitchen. It should be dark out because it's *before* sunrise, and I am guessing you have the light on your phone shining on this very page so you can read it. Do you feel like a secret agent on a mission? Or you might have a lamp on so you can read this. Or you may have turned on all the lights in your house. Anyway, I want you to go and sit somewhere you can see the sunrise and just watch it. Like, the whole thing. Just be in the moment and watch a new day dawn. There is something beautifully calming and spiritual about watching sunrise — not the morning TV show, that can be hard to watch some mornings. A sunrise is magic.

Feel free to jump in the car and drive to a headland or ride your bike to a hill or sit on your balcony or front porch or in the back paddock. Go to a park or a beach or to the edge of your lawn and sit. Take a thermos of tea if you want, and a blanket to sit on. If you have little ones and need to be at home, find a window, or wake them up so they can experience it with you. Watch how the rising of the sun transforms night into day. Feel the sun on your skin, and remember to breathe. This is a form of mindfulness. If it's raining, take an umbrella or a poncho. Don't let the rain dampen your sunrise spirit.

According to the journal *Dermato Endocrinology*, researchers have found a connection between early morning light exposure and metabolism regulation. And interestingly, the sun rises every morning, making it easy to take a purposeful moment to sit and watch something beautiful. It's a great way to start the day, before the bustle ahead kicks in. And, thanks to technology, your phone *knows* when the sun rises, so you can make this a weekly ritual if you like. Freeing yourself up in the morning can be the best way to set up your day. It gives you some peace and some space for your thoughts and a set time to set your intention for the day. A day of endless possibilities, a chance for greatness, for connection, for whatever comes across your desk. I bet you feel good, and you should. You should be proud of yourself. I'm proud of you.

Today's activity

You already nailed it by watching the sun rise, but I would also like you to reflect on this in your journal. Write about what strategy you used to get up early, and how good you feel for sticking to it. As you were up earlier than usual, you may feel an afternoon slump, so here's a friendly reminder to dip into your Sober Toolkit if you need an afternoon pick-me-up to navigate a longer than usual day without leaning on alcohol.

Two weeks into sobriety might be a good time to check in with some talk therapy with a qualified counsellor. When you consider your relationship with alcohol was such a big part of your life and your identity, it's a big shift to not have it around, and this might feel like a break-up. Unpacking these deep feelings of grief with a professional can help. The great news is that you are feeling your feelings, which is what we are meant to do with our feelings.

Day 15

Humans are hardwired for connection, and I don't just mean wi-fi. But boy do we love wi-fi! I have seen people get super angry when their wi-fi connection drops out — like throwing their phone at the wall mad. It's kind of crazy how crazy people can get when the rainbow wheel of death pops up on their laptop screen and their sacred internet seems to be somewhere off with the ~~pixels~~ pixies. Although we *think* we need wi-fi, we *need* human connection. The desire to surround ourselves with like-minded people, to find our tribe, to belong and to be heard. This is part of the human experience. Sobriety can be tough because you can feel alone. To be fair, drinking ridiculous amounts of alcohol can leave you feeling isolated too. Actively stepping away from your comfort zone of communal drinking in a bid to discover a new way of doing life can be lonely at first. So here is some validation.

You are doing a great thing.

You are doing so well.

I am so proud of you.

Yes, you might feel left out, or that you're missing out, or that you've been cut off *and not just at the bar*, but finding like-minded people is important. You don't have to trade in your old friends for a new tribe, but seeking out other activities to replace the ones fuelled by alcohol is an important part of this journey. One door closes, new ones open.

I was convinced that I *needed* alcohol to do fun things, but I was terribly mistaken. In the time I have been sober since 2015 I've done *so many* new and wonderful things I never thought I would have the courage to do. I started a podcast, I wrote a book, I eloped, I had a child, I minimised, I danced, I opened a gym, I started a business, I capsule wardrobed, I renovated a house, I studied nutrition, I went on a fitness holiday, I water-skied, I volunteered, I got chickens, I got a dog, I snowboarded and I started baking (which was problematic when I went through that Paleo phase). I have seen more, done more, thrown myself at more, with more energy and gusto than ever. And it's a direct result of my sobriety. I'm not suggesting you sign up for the CrossFit Games, but I do think exercise has its benefits. Instead of going to the pub, find a gym, a class, a physical outlet for yourself. It's helpful to plan your weeks as well, so that the odd invite to 'grab a drink this afternoon' can be easily quashed with, 'I have plans, I've got training tonight'. I discovered F45, a gym community, and I fell in love with the style of training — so much so, that I opened my own F45 studio! Not a requirement, but sobriety puts *anything is possible* as the benchmark.

> Since I quit drinking, I have written and published eight books. I've fronted a hugely successful podcast that focuses on two of my passions: women's health and empowerment. I've reached fitness goals I never would've believed possible. Instead of being a thirsty bitch, I'm a strong bitch. I have been a better friend and as a result I have made better friends. I've worked so goddamn hard at my jobs. And I've been a more present parent. Still imperfect, but definitely less shit.
>
> **Yumi Stynes — author, mum, strong bitch**

Today's activity

Let's make a mocktail! If you are entertaining, I have an alcohol-free punch approved by my 90-year-old pop, a recipe that your guests will love. And a booze-free margarita that is delish. The mocktail possibilities are endless. I prefer not to add any alcohol-free spirits. Keep it clean with the combination of fresh juices, fruits and garnish.

Cranberry bliss

Ingredients

- 100 g cranberries
- 100 mL cranberry juice
- 500 mL blood orange juice (pulp free)
- Juice of 1 lime
- 8 thin wedges of lime
- 8 thin wedges of orange
- Mint sprigs
- 600 mL sparkling apple juice

Method

Put the cranberries into a freezer container. Cover with water (by about 2.5 cm) and freeze until solid. This will create a sheet.

Mix the cranberry juice with the orange and lime juices in a large jug or punch bowl (about 1.5 L).

To serve, smash the sheet of frozen cranberries into shards and put them in the bottom of your glass along with a wedge of lime, a wedge of orange and a mint sprig. Then pour in the mixed fruit juices and top up with sparkling apple juice.

Nojito

Ingredients

- 2 lime wedges
- Flaky sea salt

(continued)

- 6 mint leaves
- 30 mL apple juice
- 20 mL lime juice
- 15 mL elderflower syrup
- crushed ice
- 40 mL soda water

Method

Wet the rim of a tumbler glass by wiping a lime wedge around the edge. Roll the rim in a small dish of flaky sea salt and tap off any excess.

Place the mint leaves in the bottom of a tall glass and press down with a muddler to extract the flavour.

Measuring with a jigger, add apple juice, lime juice and elderflower syrup to the glass.

Fill glass with crushed ice and stir.

Top up with soda water.

Day 16

Hey there sleeping beauty. Are you sleeping better? Do you always ask the person you wake up next to how they slept? Isn't what you sign up for when you marry someone, being asked every morning how you slept? And what about dreams? Dreams are such a mystery. For a couple of years in the mid noughties I suffered from night traumas, which unfortunately for me, resulted in night sweats. In the morning you'd think I'd gone for a midnight skinny dip. I was saturated. Gross. Some nights I would wake up *screaming*, which isn't fun for anyone, especially my friendly neighbours.

One night, when I lived in Adelaide, I had a terrible dream. I was trying to scream for help and I couldn't. I was trying to speak, make any sound, and I couldn't say anything. As someone who talks for a living, this is literally my worst nightmare. At the time I just passed it off as a bad dream and drank a bottle of wine, as you do — well, as I used to do and you used to, too. The night traumas have passed, thank goodness, and although I sometimes battle with anxiety (current work in progress), I have never slept better than in my sobriety. I hope you do too.

If your mind is overactive when you are trying to rest, try and write down what your dream was about. You don't need to go to a dream interpreter, but there might be things weighing on your mind. Now that you are accessing new pathways in your brain, it might be worth writing things down. Not to over-analyse, just to acknowledge the thoughts. Dream awareness can take you deeper into your subconscious and, without getting too airy-fairy, this is where you do your 'soul' work, which is the work that stays with us. So maybe, if you wake up in the middle of the night, grab your journal and write down a few things.

Today's activity

It's a journal day! Take some time today to write down:

+ five things that have improved in your life since going alcohol free

+ three people you love and why

+ one compliment to yourself.

And shout the person behind you at the café a coffee today.

It'll feel good.

Day 17

When you started this journey, did you think there would be huge vacuous gaps of time in the afternoon and into the evening that you could not fathom getting through without a drink? Did the very idea of not drinking make you feel physically ill, or extremely nervous? Did the thought of not having a drink on the weekend scare the living daylights out of you? Did you think to yourself, 'Well what on earth will I do *instead*?' Same. Glad it wasn't just me. Sometimes it's nice to be wrong! Am I right?

When you stop carrying on like a lemonhead at your local, you quickly discover how much good stuff is on offer just outside of those doors to the beer garden. At first, it is daunting. I honestly thought I would die of boredom, but it *is* possible to be sober and to thrive.

You know how I'm not a brain scientist? Well, I know one. Her name is Dr Ineka and she shared her incredible insights into how our brains work earlier in the book. Your brain has been in the consistent habit of using alcohol to entertain, engage, enlighten, relax, forget, survive, thrive, enjoy, celebrate and calm down. But now you are losing those neurons because you are not using those neurons. That's the 'use it or lose it' principal.

You are not drinking now, which means when you are happy you have been finding new ways to celebrate. When you have a rough day at work, you are finding new tools to cope and unwind. When you have a free afternoon, you are finding a new way to fill the hours by doing something productive, or good for you, or great for humankind or nice for a neighbour. The more you use these brain cells — the neurons — to fire new habits, the more new neutral pathways are created. And as we know, neurons that fire together, wire together. Change requires practising your new behaviours over and over … and over again. During the Sober 30, you will start to see your mindset change. Instead of the dread you once felt at the thought of staying sober, you will enjoy a new sense of freedom around your choice to do better because you know better.

Today's activity

It's games night! Get out the Uno, find the Monopoly, dig out a jigsaw puzzle. Spend the afternoon or early evening away from the news and playing a board game. If you are stuck for some company, Words with Friends can be a good option. Playing is such a great way to get out of your head and enjoy the company of others. My favourite games to play at home are:

+ Hide & Seek
+ Taco, Cat, Goat, Cheese, Pizza
+ any jigsaw puzzles
+ Scattergories
+ Cranium
+ Hungry Hippos
+ Twister (the water version is a great outside game too)
+ Cards Against Humanity.

Day 18

'Stick It in the Bin' was a popular segment on the *National Drive Show* I hosted. Callers would dial in to the show and tell us what they wanted to stick in the bin that week, whether it was something they were fed up with, disappointed by, annoyed about, ticked off about or frustrated by. A lot of discussion around parking fines, soy milk, forgetful husbands and the resurgence of low-rise jeans are top of mind examples.

When I initially stopped drinking, I had so much spare time on my hands. Sound familiar? Well, one day I opened my kitchen cupboard and I took everything out. I spray-and-wiped that cupboard within an inch of its life. I realised I didn't need three hand whisks, four sets of measuring cups or 17 sets of chopsticks. I even found an old electric carving knife. As I cleaned out my cupboards, I realised how much junk was just sitting in cupboards not being used, gathering dust. I divided it into three piles:

- The 'Stick It in the Bin' pile for things that were broken, rubbish, rusty, old, mouldy or unusable

- The 'Keep' pile for things that I did use, like the toaster — until I went Paleo. But then my husband started baking sourdough bread, so I am glad I kept it, along with the stick blender, slow cooker and stand mixer

- The 'Charity' pile for things that would do well in a new home with a new owner, like 15 sets of chopsticks.

Once I had the space looking less like a kitchen nightmare and more like *MasterChef*, I opened my wardrobe, and like the Lion and the Witch, I didn't exit those doors for a while. From there I discovered *The Minimalists* and my journey to living with less began. I am not a full-on minimalist, but I have adopted many of the pillars of living with less stuff. More recently I have binge watched *Marie Kondo* and am slightly obsessed with *The Home Edit*. At the end of my spontaneous spring clean, I had a capsule wardrobe, fewer roller-skates, more room and I felt light — like I could breathe, like a weight had lifted. And I have been purposeful to not refill my empty storage spaces with more junk but use intention when purchasing items. Reusing, upcycling, op-shopping, freaking antiquing and giving away are all principles for spending less on less and giving things a new life. It's not to say that we can't have nice things. I didn't cancel Netflix or give away my car, but I did toss the things that were cluttering up my cupboards and gathering dust in the drawers. I kept and organised the sentimental things, and I turned my home — eventually, over time — into a functional living space that I love.

Today's activity

Do I need to spell it out for you? Find a drawer. Clear it out and see how it feels. But start small. One draw, one cupboard, one room at a time.

Highly recommended resources for this project include:

- The Minimilists — books, docos, essays, podcast — www.theminimilists.com
- Marie Kondo — Netflix series
- The Home Edit — Netflix series, Instagram @thehomedit
- The Art of Decluttering — podcast

Day 19

Oh hey, you look great today!

Some people around you can get a bit weird about your choice to go sober. We are creatures of habit, and if someone is going to dare to do something wildly differently from the popular choice, then there seems to be immediate opposition.

Oh, why are you doing that? (Eye roll)

Why would you bother? (Shrug)

Everyone else is drinking. (Sigh!)

How long will that last? (Smirk)

We like our comfort zones. They feel nice: like snuggling into a boyfriend pillow on a rainy weekend (so I've heard). The living part of life starts just outside and slightly to the left of your comfort zone. What helped me get my head around the big factor of 'other humans' — because, let's face it, other humans are unavoidable — was the realisation that *my* choice held up a mirror to *their* choices. The way people respond is very revealing. It says everything about them and very little about you. If someone is negative about your sobriety, it could be too challenging for them to comprehend for themselves. A reaction of shock, disappointment and sometimes disbelief is potentially the truth of their own narrative around alcohol. This is their discomfort with themselves, not you. So, do as Adele suggests and go easy on them:

- *Be compassionate.* Some people will simply not understand the truth bomb you've exploded into your own life, and that's okay, you can be kind.

- *Be honest.* Ask for the support you need and remind the person you are not after their approval.

- *Be okay about walking away* if you find yourself in a situation that just feels too peer-pressure-y.

Today's activity

Ground down. Find a quiet place today and sit for 10 minutes. Spend some quality time with you. The more time you spend away from screens, other people, outside noise, bingeing on TV, scrolling through Insta and other distractions, the more you can say 'hi' to you. If you can find a quiet spot — a café courtyard, a waterfall, a cosy nook, a park, a garden — sit somewhere quiet, listen to nature and chill. Let the souls of your feet or palms of your hands touch the earth. This is called grounding. Fans of grounding include me, Gwyneth Paltrow and Sally Fitzgibbons.

Day 20

I think that when I first drank as a teen it was about dealing with social anxiety. I was trying to fit in. But when I started in a band, I realised I didn't need to fit in. Alcohol was just a mask, and it wasn't going to send me in a good direction long term.
Janet English — Spiderbait, rockstar, sober

The concert will play, the show will go on, the night will come to an end and the fireworks will look pretty and not show up so well in photos. The event will happen, whether you get there and get drunk or not. One of my biggest fears deciding to go alcohol free was how many events and cool parties I'd miss. I thought I loved being around people in social environments. Remember this was in a season of life when I was convinced I was an extroverted personality type and somewhat of a social butterfly. It turns out I am an introverted extrovert and much prefer being at home and having quiet nights in. The alcohol became my crutch to cope with the anxiety my mismatched personality type and career choice presented. A big surprise for me was the relief I found in sobriety. I didn't need to keep up appearances anymore. I could honour my truth and be as low key as I wanted. I could stay in. Oh, the relief. Fear is just dumb. Fear is an unpleasant emotion caused by the threat of danger, pain or harm. And when you have been so used to drinking in social settings or to cope with your life choices, the idea of living without alcohol is fear inducing. It feels like a threat.

The way our upside-down society is constructed, you have been conditioned to become afraid of what people will say if you do something new, or don't do something everyone else is doing — even if it isn't working for you. And let's be clear, drinking hasn't been working for you. It didn't work for me either. When I accepted the party could go on without me, I felt a profound sense of relief. I could go if I wanted, be in control, drive home and enjoy the next day, or skip it all together. Either way, it was my empowered choice. The irrational fears I had of becoming *boring*, or not having *any* fun due to my sobriety, were just false fears. I had given too much power to 'the night out', which was robbing me of a harmonious life. When you let go of your need to be at the party, the party happens, and you will find a peaceful way to create the life you want to live.

Today's activity

Go on a picnic today! A picnic is the ultimate sobriety hack. It is a daytime activity that doesn't require any alcohol. It's social, easy to pack up, it's an outside activity and it's completely appropriate to leave before the sun sets. When I stopped drinking, I did start socialising at a different hour and in a different way, and picnics became my new favourite way to spend time with friends and family. Buy a reflex tennis set, a portable BBQ, a frisbee or some playing cards. Invest in a Moroccan picnic rug and create the ultimate picnic. Go to town on some Tupperware, a grazing board and fruit platters that matter. Take a thermos of tea and stacks of sparkling water.

Day 21

It takes 21 days to change a habit. Or does it? The 21-day theory of habit change isn't exactly what it's been pitched as. It's needed a bit of a rebrand. Let me explain. Dr Maxwell Maltz's work on self-image observed changes were adapted to in 'a minimum of about 21 days'. His observations were around patients receiving plastic surgery and how long it would take for the patient to get used to seeing their new face. These experiences were observational, and the takeaway was a pattern of about 21 days to adjust to a new situation. A later study conducted by University College of London health psychology researcher Phillippa Lally examined the habits of 96 people over a 12-week period. Not a huge sample size, but still valid. Each person chose one new habit for a 12-week reporting period. Everything from 'drinking a bottle of water with lunch', to 'running for 15 minutes before dinner'. Researchers concluded on average it takes more than two months before a new behaviour becomes automatic — 66 days to be exact. And this can vary widely depending on the behaviour, the person and the circumstances. In Lally's study, it took anywhere from 18 days to 254 days for people to form a new habit. In saying that, you've got to start somewhere, right? And 30 days is a good goal to begin the rewiring process — and you, my friend, are adjusting your behaviour, so good for you!

Today's activity

Get lost. Go somewhere you have never been before. A trampoline park, that new pop-up store, an art gallery, a museum, a night market, a carnival, a dance class, a cooking class, a park, a footy field, a hike, a trail, a headland, a mountain, an open road, a meeting, a meet-up, a restaurant, a café, a quiet corner of nature off the beaten track, a concert, a creek, a lake, a bakery — anywhere, but somewhere new. Be somewhere you've never been before.

Day 22

So, a bit of background on me: before I found my fitness religion at F45, I was a fad diet junkie and a fitness trend enthusiast. I did it all. Every kind of boot camp, yoga trend, fitness thing, expert diet, celebrity-endorsed eating plan. You name it. I did it. And, to keep you up to speed, I now do a daily yoga practice and have ditched the high-intensity stuff. A combination of squeaky knees and migraines had me switch up my movement mantra. Anyway, whenever I was on the lemon detox, beetroot, cabbage soup, South Beach, Atkins, blood-type, Zone, juice only, ballerina tea or potato diet, I noticed I would crave the very thing I was depriving myself of. I guess it's mind over matter — or is it the way that it shatters that matters? Oh nope, that was a Violet Crumble ad. I could never tell the difference between a Violet Crumble and a Crunchie: that was a real head scratcher in my early teens ...

So, cravings.

Cravings. Yeah, for some reason, our brains seem to focus on the one thing we can't have rather than celebrating the hundreds (well, maybe not so much on the beetroot diet) *available* options. This is the same for drinking alcohol. So, what can you do when a little craving pops up?

Find a good alternative. Have a good alternative on standby to quash that little craving when it pops up. Here are some suggestions:

- sparkling mineral water

- regular filtered water

- no-alcohol ginger beer

- kombucha

- a thermos of tea

- fresh juice

- cucumber water

- a smoothie.

Today's activity

DIY. Make something from scratch. A dinner, a dessert, a cake, a cookie, a table, a bookshelf, a website, a drawing, a Lego tower, a go-kart. Be as simple or elaborate as you care to be. There is something satisfying about starting at the beginning with your bare hands and, with some time and a few implements, creating something.

Day 23

Time to start looking ahead.

The future looks bright.

Sobriety is my superpower. You want to know why? I can't screw it up. It's zero drinks of alcohol for me. End of discussion. The line is drawn, the boundary is clear and this works me for. It's easy now because it's learnt behaviour. I am clear on my intention each day to be sober. I once read a quote — okay, to be fair, it was most likely a pin on Pinterest — and it said, 'Don't dwell on the good old days; they weren't that good'. And I thought *Screw you Mr. My* good old days were awesome! Did you see my sense of flair and fashion? Did you see me ride the heights of success? Did you see my media career skyrocket?

Deep down, however, the common thread was that I was always drinking. Yes, I have some great stories and I met a tonne of famous people, and yes, I was a success, but I wasn't connected to myself. I was unable to experience the full measure of life because I was leaning on alcohol to get me through. I reflect fondly on those days when my life looked very different. I appreciate it for what it was, and I am grateful for the experiences, but I am so thankful to have chosen a new path. You may have had the best night ever (and forgotten most of it), but now you can have the best life ever — a life made up of great days. And your best days are ahead, my friend. A future without alcohol may seem intimidating still, but there is an amazing community of people who have walked through this already, so get connected into a community of like-minded people and share your sobriety story so far. Hopefully when you look ahead you'll see endless possibilities and good vibes only.

Today's activity

Get online. Find an online platform, a hub, a safe place to share your story and feel empowered by others who are walking the path alongside you. Maybe you want to write a blog or put up a social post about your experience so far. You will find encouragement flows towards you. Have a dig around for like-minded people. Reach out and share your thoughts and find someone to encourage on their journey as you get encouraged on yours.

Day 24

Morning blossom, did you spring out of bed today? Probably not. No-one really does that, do they? I'm guessing you hit snooze a couple of times and ran late to work and so now you're reading this in your lunchbreak. Just a guess. Today, with your newfound clarity, you can get a head start on evaluating your legacy. How do you feel about continuing this journey of self-acceptance, self-love and learning? At our core, I think we know the truth. Learning to trust your gut is a life skill that will serve you well. The more you rely on it, the louder it will direct you. I call it our spiritual GPS. There are times when I went against my gut and realised, in the aftermath of that choice, I knew what to do but I didn't listen. Listening to your internal voice will guide you towards better choices — not necessary the *easy* choice, but the better one. And using your inner guide is like building a muscle: the more you use it, the stronger it gets. Ultimately, it's you who makes your own choices, and our choices create our life experience. Today's footprint is tomorrow's legacy, and the good choices that you are making today are setting you up for a brighter tomorrow. You are now living in an awakened and empowered reality. Take some time to think about, and position yourself for the long game.

Today's activity

Do something selfless to make someone else have a better day. It will fill you up! And I encourage you to do it regularly. Buying a round at the bar doesn't count. Nice try though. You could:

- bake cookies for your colleagues
- volunteer your time
- cook a meal and drop it on a friend's doorstep
- visit your elderly relatives or neighbour
- babysit your friends' rowdy kids so they can have a date night
- give away that jacket
- give an old friend a call
- take someone out for lunch
- buy someone a bunch of flowers
- send a complimentary email of praise
- say thank you
- smile at a stranger
- shout someone a hashbrown.

Day 25

How good are you feeling? Yeah, I thought so. Mental clarity feels so good. Do you feel like you have a new lens that you're looking through? I did. It was about day 25 when things shifted for me. I stopped thinking about not having a drink, and I experienced a paradigm shift (the Oxford dictionary defines a paradigm shift as a great and important change in the way something is done or thought about).

At first, the shift happened with my fitness training. I had always worked out, even at the height of my drinking behaviour. I did aerobics for school sport. I was always, forever and ever (Amen) on my way to training. Either at the gym, or to bootcamp, dance class, yoga, boxing. Like I said, keeping fit has always been a part of my world, even when I was boozing it up.

However, before giving up alcohol, my motivation for fitness was 'I have to work out so I won't put on weight'. My motivation was to avoid an outcome of being too big for my height, or the wrong shape or size for my job, but this changed when I stopped drinking. I reframed my motivation for working out as working towards a goal, rather than to avoid an outcome. My mental shift became, 'I want to work out to discover my healthiest self'. See the difference? Be the difference.

When my thinking about fitness shifted dramatically, so did my thinking about many things. Similarly, with sobriety it shifted from 'a time to reflect on my drinking behaviour' to 'I want to see how much greater this can get'. Try and find the fuel to drive you towards what you want or want to become.

Today's activity

Journal it out. Write about the person who started this journey 25 days ago:

- How you felt
- How you made decisions
- How you looked at life
- How you looked
- What your driver was.

Then write about how you feel today — the person who is starring in this story:

- How do you feel?
- How are you making decisions?
- What is your overall sense about your life?
- How do you look?
- What is sparking joy for you?

See the difference?

Day 26

Martin Luther King Jr said, 'Faith is taking the first step even when you don't see the whole staircase.'

Do you have faith in yourself? I hope by now you have a renewed sense of faith in your own abilities. You are kicking ass in this journey. Faith is complete trust in someone or something; it's an ability to hope for the things unseen. Faith is not a feeling. It's a state of mind, it's a lack of self-doubt. Is there a voice — or if you're like me, many voices — in your head telling you you're not good enough, brave enough, strong enough? Or that you will fail? This is the voice that taunts you when you set out to do a new thing. The one that criticises you when things are difficult. Self-doubt is greedy. It can devour confidence, remove logic and reason from your mind and steal happiness from your heart, leaving you with fear and insecurity. I am giving you permission to tell that voice to be quiet. Turn it down. Fade it out. Find the good voice, the encourager, your biggest fan. Your support cheering you on from the sidelines. Give *that* voice the platform, the space in your head and the microphone in your mind. Hold onto the faith that you are capable of sobriety. You are doing it. See? Look at you go. You took the first step in sobriety, and you have kept your pace. Consistency is the key, and as you keep walking in sobriety, you can lean on the faith in yourself that you can do this, you can keep going, you can trust yourself again. The glory comes not from not falling, but from rising again. This sobriety journey is an active lesson in how we pick ourselves up, dust ourselves off, keep the faith and keep going.

Today's activity

Go for a walk today and take your earbuds. Listen to something inspiring or just plain darn hilarious.

My top podcast recommendations for a casual stroll in your free time include:

+ *Super Soul Conversations*, Oprah

+ *We Can Do Hard Things*, Glennon Doyle

+ *Unlocking Us*, Brené Brown

+ *Do You F***ing Mind*, Alexis Fernandez

+ *The Tony Robbins Podcast*

+ *Serial*, Sarah Koenig

+ *Making* series, WBEZ Chicago

+ *Armchair Expert*

+ *The Michelle Obama Podcast*

+ *Smartless*, Jason Bateman, Will Arnett and Sean Hayes

+ *Last Drinks*, Maz Compton

+ *Maz & Matty*.

Day 27

There is a remarkable difference between being self-aware and being self-obsessed. Being self-aware is a gift and it's a challenge. In today's busy as a badge of honour society there are no fewer than two trillion distractions from work, family and self. Just a casual observation: it is quite normal to be very focused on status updates, follower checks, replies, likes and virality. Not to say that any of these things are bad. They can absolutely be a part of a healthy self-profile, but let's turn the focus on being self-aware. Being self-aware is more about being observant, calculated, cautious and kind. The difference? Obsession is externalised; awareness is internalised. The conscious knowledge of one's own character, feelings and desires is the art of self-awareness and when you are self-aware, you can see the imprint you have on others. Here are some simple tips to keep you self-aware, not self-obsessed:

- *Own your phone.* Be in control of what messages get to you and what isn't important. Mute the emails and push notifications that come soaring your way. Each time you stop to respond to a text or a tweet, you are pulling yourself away from the task in front of you. Turn off your phone for one full day a week and after 7 pm every night. Leave your work at work. Set healthy boundaries around your screen time and online engagements.

- *Dedicate some 'me' time.* Spend enough time alone to become comfortable with your own company. Want a big fat haloumi burger on your lunchbreak but can't find a co-worker to go with? Go it alone. Allow yourself to be comfortable with just you and that amazing haloumi burger. Be confident you can do things by yourself.

- *Breathe mindfully.* Sit with good posture, practise a steady breath and let thoughts escape your mind. A simple mindfulness exercise for just 10 minutes may surprise you with its calming effect.

- *Be productive.* Set your mind to the task at hand and have a threshold of excellence. In your work, home and play. Do things 100 per cent. Full out.

Self-awareness is about leading your own life in a meaningful and impactful manner. It's about enjoying the little things, finding good in the bad and ultimately focusing on what brings you joy.

Today's activity

Give yourself a physical treat. Run a bath, have a foot spa, do a facial, book a massage; get a neck rub, a leg rub or a body scrub; lie with your lower back on a foam roller or a rolled-up towel. Give yourself half an hour to chill and unwind today. You deserve it.

Day 28

Well, well, well, it's been a short month and you are sober and thriving. Good for you. So, it's taken me this entire month to drum up the courage to share a personal story. It involves my husband. Most of the stories in this book are just about me because I like to keep my private life, well, private. So I don't talk too much about my wonderful mini human, or my incredible husband, but this story is worth sharing. My husband, Glen, is a builder by trade. He is also sober. One afternoon in the first year I stopped drinking I got home earlier than expected, not expecting Glen to be home earlier than expected too. When Glen is on the tools, his days are physically tough, and then he has to deal with me — emotionally tough. I am a super empath and need to debrief a lot. I came swooning through the door like something out of *Absolutely Fabulous* — to be fair I am more *Miss Congeniality* when I swan into a room. Anyway, Glen was sitting on the couch watching something on his laptop. As he saw me enter the room, he slammed the laptop shut. I freaked out.

Why is he home?

What was he watching?

Why are my socks on the floor?

I asked, very calmly — to be fair it was probably snappier than calm — 'What are you doing home?'

There was a moment of awkward silence and then he replied, 'I finished work early and I'm watching a French dude make sourdough on his YouTube channel.'

You see, we had watched a Netflix series, *Cooked*, the week before. It's excellent, and one of the episodes was about bread. The bread we buy in the supermarket can have up to 27 ingredients, most of them unpronounceable. The documentary explained bread is just three simple ingredients: flour, water and salt. I have argued that there are four ingredients if you include air (for the fermenting process). Glen was inspired to master sourdough. This was pre-pandemic, mind you. He was ahead of his time. And so, that afternoon he was watching a French dude on YouTube explain the process of sourdough breadmaking.

Today's activity

Watch YouTube on your laptop, and when your partner gets home, see the look of potential fear on their face...no, I'm kidding.

Get baking! It's a lost skill and we need to bring it back. Like how the boys brought Backstreet back and how Katie Holmes is still trying to bring back 1990s fashion.

Here are some suggestions off the top of my chef's hat:

+ cupcakes
+ cookies
+ crumble
+ bread (obvs)
+ shortbread
+ honey joys
+ muesli slice
+ house-made granola

- slow cooker brownies
- chocolate zucchini loaf
- banana bread
- carrot cake muffins
- the 'I Quit Sugar' lime cheesecake
- grown-ups rocky road.

Day 29

What a remarkable achievement. You are totally doing life, doing it well and doing it sober! You know what you might feel like doing today? Having a drink. Why? Because you are almost at the end of the commitment you made to see this thing through and somehow when you get a handle on things it seems like a fair reward to take your foot off the gas and give yourself a break and have a drink.

Please don't do that.

That's not a good idea. Can I tell you why? You don't need a drink. You can function without it. You know that alcohol is carcinogenic; you know it's only going to mess with your body function, your brain function and your emotions. You know it doesn't help any situation you're facing. You know it doesn't help you relax, you know it's not a positive reward, you know it will leave you feeling empty. You know all this. So, trust yourself to get through today without a drink. If you feel like celebrating, refer to your Sober Toolkit and find ways to celebrate that are empowering, that will lift you up and carry you through and reinforce the good decisions you have made about being sober.

Today's activity

Tea is the most popular beverage in the world, equalling all other liquids including coffee, chocolate, soft drinks and alcohol *combined*. So, let's have a party — a tea party! You might be missing your bottle of empty calories, but there are so many better drink options out there. I have barrels, bags and buckets of tea in my pantry, all beautifully labelled in pantry-porn-style containers with bamboo lids. *The Home Edit* girls would be so proud of me. The pantry overhaul was one of my most favourite sobriety activities! I love clearing out cupboards and I love a cuppa tea. There is something wholesome and therapeutic about tea. Try becoming a tea nut, you peanut. Biscuits are optional, but my personal recommendation with an English Breakfast tea is a Digestive biscuit.

Teas to try

+ Yorkshire tea with a dash of milk

+ Green tea: 80°C is the perfect temperature

+ Oolong tea

+ Bancha tea

+ Matcha Green latte

+ Yerba Mate

+ Liquorice tea

+ Japanese green tea

+ Masala Chai on almond milk

+ Apple Turkish tea

+ Iced tea, with a slice of lemon

+ Strawberry iced tea

+ Earl Grey latte

+ London Fog

+ Ginger tea

+ Honey and lemon tea.

Day 30

Hey you:

- You look better.
- You feel better.
- Your mind is clearer.
- Your body is functioning better.
- Your brain is sharper.
- Your creativity has been unleashed.
- You have stood up to resistance.
- Your hair is thicker.
- Your nails are stronger.
- Your eyes are clearer.
- Your pockets are heavier.
- You're more self-aware.
- Your anxiety is subsiding.
- You are more active.
- You have more energy.
- You feel smarter.
- You are stronger.
- You are lighter.

- You are more patient.

- You are nicer.

- You are calmer.

You are welcome!

Today's activity

Take a selfie. Compare it to the selfie you took on day 1.

I know you feel good, so do some journalling today. What are you grateful for? I am grateful for you.

Congratulations. You did something that you thought you couldn't (but I knew you could). You are amazing. You are sober and thriving. Let's get through today and then we can debrief. You have set yourself apart and stood out from the crowd for the right reason — go you! You have steadily, day by day, climbed to the top of a mountain and now it's up to you to stay there and enjoy the view. Enjoy today. Stay sober. Feel proud. Your better, healthier, happier, lighter and brighter, sober self is here because you created the space for sobriety.

Bonus activity

Find a beautiful way to celebrate your first sober month.

Final words

I feel like we understand each other. I have walked along this very same path, and I kept going. And I hope you do too. The freedom and the fun I have found in my daily sobriety has been life changing for me and I hope you feel the same way. This new freedom that you have unlocked can be an important start for changing other behaviours and parts of your life. Amazing! You feel so good, right? So why would you go back to a behaviour that you know will lead you away from this empowerment and goodness? It can be easy to think you're done. You did 30 days and that's good enough, and it is great.

I think it's amazing what you have walked through, but you can keep going. An entire season of life, three months or a year in sobriety will be the best way to reward yourself for starting this journey. Keep going. You know alcohol and its impact is only going to mess up all the work you've done. You have now had a taste of sobriety and you know it's so satiating. We are all on the journey to betterment. It's endless if you are open to consistently being moulded into a better you. You have rediscovered old loves, found new strength, saved time, saved money and you've discovered a new way to do life. This new you can impact many other areas of your life. You used to use alcohol to cope, which would warp your perspective, and your load felt heavy. But now you know the truth: you can do life, every bit of it, without alcohol. You have the tools in your toolkit, and over the past month you have proven to yourself you can be sober and thrive. All it takes is one simple choice at a time. A decision to live without alcohol is a decision for you — for your health and for your future best self.

My ultimate wish for you is to continue towards a version of you who is vibrant, healthy and whole. A version of you who tackles tough roads with grace and style, who rises to the challenge with inner might and who becomes a light to others.

Remember, sweet friend: you have a choice, always.

You only get one day once. Make it beautiful.

And finally, you are meant to be here. Now go and be sober and thrive.

All my love and soda waters.

Maz Compton
Alcohol free since 2015

Additional resources

Throughout this book are snippets of some of the wonderful conversations I have had on the *Last Drinks* podcast. If you would like to listen to the complete conversations and hear the whole stories, please refer to the episode guide below. You can listen to *Last Drinks* wherever you get your podcasts, and a new episode is published each week. Subscribe so you don't miss an episode and follow @lastdrinkspod to stay up to date.

Janet English, Spiderbait, Episode 1

My Sobriety Superpower, Episode 5

Rob Mills, Entertainer, Episode 6

Safeguarding Your Sobriety, Episode 7

Fiona Redding, The Happiness Hunter, Episode 10

Sobriety Is Self-Care, Episode 11

Irene Falcone, Founder, Sans Drinks, Episode 12

Bex Weller, Founder, Sexy Sobriety, Episode 14

Osher Günsberg, TV and Podcast Host, Episode 16

Dr Buddhi Lokuge, Addiction Expert, Episodes 17 and 19

Mindful Drinking, Episodes 20 and 21

Libby McMichael, Yoga Teacher, Episode 22

Belle Robertson, Sober Coach, Episode 28

Yumi Stynes, Media Personality, Episode 29

Jay Mueller, Podcast Producer, Episode 30

Blair Sharp, The Sobriety Activist, Episode 33

David Campbell, TV Host, Episode 34

Heidi Anderson, PR Queen, Episode 36

Action Alexa, Motivation/Fitness Expert, Episode 37

Maz Compton, Author, Podcast Host, Episode 40

Casey Davidson, Sobriety Coach, Episode 44

Kathryn Elliott, Breast Cancer Survivor, Episode 46

Dr Ineka Whiteman, Neuroscientist, Episode 47

How to Celebrate Sober, Episode 50

Dr Matt Agnew, scientist Episode 52

Further resources

Here is a list of resources you may find useful during your journey in sobriety.

Counselling

Beyond Blue: 1300 22 46 36

- www.beyondblue.org.au/get-support/talk-to-a-counsellor
- www.beyondblue.org.au/support-service/chat

Crisis support

Lifeline: 13 11 14

- www.lifeline.org.au

Helpful hashtags

#sobriety

#lastdrinks

#alcoholfreeliving

#sobercurious

#soberliving

Connect with Maz

www.mazcompton.com

@mazcompton on Instagram and Facebook

@lastdrinkspod on Instagram

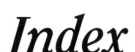

Index